WONDERS
of a single dose
IN
HOMOEOPATHY

D1715810

WONDERS
of
A SINGLE DOSE
in
HOMEOPATHY

Dr. K.D. Kanodia

Revised Second Edition

B. JAIN PUBLISHERS (P) LTD.
USA – Europe – India

WONDERS OF A SINGLE DOSE IN HOMEOPATHY

First Edition: 1989
Second Revised and Enlarged Edition: 2008
3rd Impression: 2014

All rights reserved. No part of this book may be reproduced, stored in a retrieval system or transmitted, in any form or by any means, mechanical, photocopying, recording or otherwise, without any prior written permission of the publisher.

© with the publisher

Published by Kuldeep Jain for
B. JAIN PUBLISHERS (P) LTD.
1921/10, Chuna Mandi, Paharganj, New Delhi 110 055 (INDIA)
Tel.: +91-11-4567 1000   Fax: +91-11-4567 1010
Email: info@bjain.com   Website: **www.bjain.com**

Printed in India by
J.J. Offset Printers

ISBN: 978-81-319-0308-7

PREFACE TO FIRST EDITION

Since 1810, when the *natural law of healing* was brought to light by **Dr. Samuel Christian Fredrick Hahnemann**, the science of homeopathy (*Similia Similibus Curentur-likes are cured by likes*) has much advanced.

Basically, homeopathy **restores the body** to health by **stimulating the healing forces within the body.**

This volume of the compilation is to highlight the achievements by renowned physicians of the world; to create a feeling of confidence and surety of results in this system; to acquaint the people and profession about the wonders of the drug in potency; and to impress upon all, that it is the **quickest and the safest system** of restoring health.

Homeopathy studies the plant life, animal life and the metals with all the aspects and background and establishes **a relation to individual human life in particular condition.** This co-relation and co-incidence of symptoms is the key note of homeopathy.

A pathologist examines a sick person from head to foot and finds no proof of sickness. And still the person under examination complains that he has **a long list of sufferings. He has no refreshing sleep, has aches and pains, and various discomforts, always perplexed, worried and uneasy.**

Homeopathy studies these *symptoms* which are the **language of nature and that they indicate and focus the internal sickness leading to some major disaster.**

The stage of clear diagnosis comes when the breakdown occurs, the vital force gives way and you have consumption, fatty degeneration of heart or cirrhosis of liver and so on.

One has to agree that the patient is **sick before** the localisation of the diseases.

Dr. J.T. Kent observes, "Under **traditional methods**, it is necessary that a diagnosis be made before the treatment can be settled, but in most cases, the **diagnosis cannot be made until results of the disease have rendered the patient incurable."**

So we need to study the internal and the external man separately. The man feels, sees, tastes, hears, thinks and lives as also he wills and understands. The body is the house **where the internal man resides.** To illustrate, *Dr. James Tyler Kent says, "One who is suffering from conscience, does not need a surgeon, but a priest. He, who has a lacerated wound, or a broken bone or deformities, has need of a surgeon. If his tooth must come out, he must have a surgeon dentist. If the physician acts also as a surgeon, he should stitch up a wound, but should not burn out an ulcer with nitrate of silver."*

When "signs and symptoms are present, the physician is needed, because these come from **interior to exterior."**

Our aim should be to discriminate and remove the external causes and turn into order, **internal disorders.**

For example, a patient comes to us with a bad food **habit** and if we keep on giving him *Nux vomica*, it is not advisable.

"Vicious habits, bad living, living in dampness are **externals** and must be removed. When a man avoids these externals, is cleanly, carefully chooses his food, and has a

iv

comfortable home, and **is still miserable,** he must be treated **from within."**

A physician has to strengthen the **vital force,** increase resistance, **decrease the susceptibility** and allow the nature to heal the patient perfectly and soundly.

There are wrong notions that **homeopathy** is not very **quick,** it is **not suitable** for all occasions, it is **not useful** as a palliative and that it requires **a long time** to cure. It is not so, **not at all so.**

The disappointments occur only **when we are out of the track. A homeopath seeks to establish a harmony and co-incidence between the language of ailments and the language of drug action.** He has to be conscious of the drug properties with regard to their reaction on a healthy body in **all aspects,** i.e. physical, emotional and mental which include feelings, sensations, cravings, aversions, ameliorations, aggravations, time, weather conditions, temperaments etc. **Both the similars** when meet together, neutralize the disease conditions, and at the same time help the resistance to increase its power against susceptibility to disease forces.

In practice, we find sometime, such situations when either the symptoms are not so very clear in their indications or if they are clear, the **drugs do not react.** Our masters have **covered most of such situations** with directions to handle them. But these require to be arranged and illustrated in full context to be made more useful to the people and profession. **This shall be the subject matter of subsequent volumes.**

Dr. K.D. Kanodia
A-213, Kewal Park
Azadpur, Delhi-33
Ph.: 91-11-27675367, 27671169

v

PREFACE TO REVISED SECOND EDITION

TALES OF WONDERS IN HOMEOPATHY

The **PIONEERS** of homeopathy have mentioned at every step that a dose of homeopathic medicine does wonders. They speak of their experiences about curing even **twenty years old Asthma** and such other chronic cases with one dose!

Does it still happens in such cases!

Then, we find in the literature at various places that the pioneers gave a series of medicines **based on Symptoms** with no results, and later on, the dose of a particular remedy was given which worked wonders!

Was it simply hit and miss!

Dr. Hahnemann - a man of conscience - admitted that, he could not cure a single chronic case even with the **best selected** remedies on the basis of symptoms available with him. And **then** he narrated the cure of 183 cases of Typhus - with *Bryonia* and *Rhus tox.* in alternation - in all cases without a single **failure;** even when all these cases **differed** in their symptoms, so much so that almost all the patients appeared apparently to be **suffering from different diseases!**

Is there anything more important than symptoms!

At places, it has been told that a single symptom led the physician to reach the right remedy; and at other occasions, a number of matching symptoms kept them in confusion and despair.

Is there anything wrong in our approach to the Science!

Dr. Hahnemann spoke of 'near specifics' in homeopathy which worked almost with surety. It seems that his mind could **foresee** the distant future where confusion was **likely** to prevail, and finding more 'specifics' could be a boon.

Why was this trend not allowed to develop!

Dr. Kent forcefully proclaimed that the system **is yet not** capable of curing diseases like **Cancer and Consumption,** and those who boast of curing these should be seen with suspicion!

What about our claims today!

Dr. Kent acquainted us with the **danger** of **Homeopathic** remedies if **wrongly used.** He considered them even most dangerous on earth at times.

Was his warning highlighted and analysed further!

Dr. Nash laid too much or **sole emphasis** on symptoms and even ignored the importance of **inimicals.** He claimed of curing innumerable cases (chronic and difficult) in his life.

Did he conceal some other factor which led to his cures!

Dr. Nash recommended to use **vegetable** based remedies first and then to use **mineral or animal** based.

Was this formula further worked out!

Dr. Kent declared some remedies as **dangerous** in certain **stages** of diseases.

Has this been further investigated!

Dr. Kent also referred about, some **"patch up remedies"** that were considered to be safe in certain **conditions and stages.**

Have we highlighted these for further research!

Dr. Burnett was very much **disappointed** with the prevailing practice during his time. He could not get any favourable results in **skin** diseases. He touched **new horizons** by applying new methods in using *Thuja* and *Bacillinum*. He also applied **ladder system** i.e. giving one medicine after the other to cover various aspects **step by step.**

Have people appreciated his experiences!

There was a report in a journal that **a case** was referred to 700 Homeopathic Physicians and they all gave **different prescriptions** for the case.

Is something being done for such chaos in the system!

Dr. Hahnemann wanted homeopathy to be a **mathematical science** in certainty where there is only **one straight line** between two given points.

Are his dreams being ignored!

Homeopathy started with **provings** of single medicines in potency on conscious, educated and healthy **human beings**. Now compounds and mixtures are being introduced with remarks on them as **"approved"** and used in material doses.

Should we reconcile to the change!

Dr. M.L. Tyler tried to draw homeopathy nearer to **Astrology**. She mentions in her *Bryonia* chapter of *'Drug Pictures'* that if one can find **9 symptoms** in a patient pertaining to *Bryonia*, she can **bet favourable** results. One has simply **to advertise** for such a patient. It is like searching for **a horoscope** where certain planets are housed at certain places, and even then **uncertainty prevails**.

Has this drawn attention of Conscientious homeopaths!

Dr. Kent was **jeered at** by people in his time for the system he adopted. His individual success in homeopathy had no mass appreciation.

Are we doing something to make the system develop as a science!

Homeopathy was introduced as a science. Our pioneers declared it as a **perfect Science**. Then **gradually** it was converted to an **Art** - where every individual has his **own display**. Further, then, it has started being treated as a **Religion** and the Homeopaths are asked to **unite** and show their strength to get benefits. **Dr. Hahnemann** is being worshipped and garlanded, but **his principles are being thrown aside**.

Is it not necessary to save the 'Pathy' from disaster ahead!

In the **subsequent** newly added chapters of revised and enlarged volume, we shall **discuss** the ways, whereby

(i) homeopathy can **revive** its glory of showing wonders again,

(ii) **analysing** the **basic factors** responsible for the faded and disappointing results at present, and

(iii) **reasons** for its derailment from the principles on which it was established.

Dr. K.D. KANODIA

A-213, Kewal Park
Azadpur, Delhi-33
August 28, 2006

x

PUBLISHER'S NOTE

Millions of pearls of wisdom are scattered over in the ocean of knowledge imparted by the pioneers of homeopathy. Nothing is original except the **provings of drugs** and their symptoms brought to light from time to time as also the **clinical experiences** highlighted by the master minds.

The requirement of the time is to assemble the technicalities in a way that the pearls become useful as ornaments and the science can be used on a wider scale by:

(a) the busy physicians

(b) the learners, and

(c) the educated masses who can study, understand and realise the blessings showered upon the human race by the originator of this science.

The author's present work is a milestone in this direction and we feel confident that this will render the science more interesting to study, more practical to practice and more certain and fast for the results expected.

KULDEEP JAIN
MD, B. Jain Publishers (P) Ltd.

ABOUT THE AUTHOR

Dr. K.D. Kanodia

Birth: Sept. 8, 1930

Education: Patna and Punjab Universities

Academic profile: BA (Hons.) MDSH, ND, DI Hom (The British Institute of Hom., London) MRSH (London).

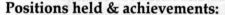

Positions held & achievements:

- Author of about two dozen books on homeopathy, social and religious aspects.

- Edited monthly organ of Delhi Hom. Med. Association, New Delhi.

- Life member - DHMA New Delhi, IIPA New Delhi, Indian Red Cross Delhi, Accident Relief Society (Regd.) Delhi, etc.

- Member - Internatonal Hom. League, Geneva, Asian Hom. Medical League, Trivandrum.

- Recipient, Appreciation Award in Homeopath from Board of Hom. System of Med., Delhi.

- Considerable Research Work done in Homeopathy and Ayurveda.

- Serving Homeopathy through Charitable Dispensaries and Renowned Hospitals.

- Appreciations from people of the country and abroad and also the State Chief Ministers, Governers, Vice Chancellors and Schloars of repute.

BOOKS BY THE SAME AUTHOR

- ☞ The Homeopathic Physicians's Quick Prescriber, 2nd Edition
- ☞ Homeopathic Chalisa, Hindi, 2nd Edition
- ☞ Rasoi Chalisa, Hindi, 2nd Edition
- ☞ 250 years of Homeopathy, 2nd Edition
- ☞ Secrets of Sure and Quick Results, 2nd Edition
- ☞ Augmented Supplement of Dr. W. Boericke's Materia Medica, 2nd Edition
- ☞ The Concepts of Miasms in Homeopathy and New Era, 2nd Edition
- ☞ Some Essential References in Repertory, 2nd Edition
- ☞ A Table Talk in Homeopathy, 2nd Edition
- ☞ Look Busy do Nothing, Hindi, 2nd Edition
- ☞ A Concise Materia Medica of Mental Symptoms in Homeopathy, 2nd Edition
- ☞ Life Saving Drugs in Homeopathy
- ☞ Advanced Homeopathy
- ☞ Quick Prescriber in Homeopathy
- ☞ Drug Zones in Homeopathy
- ☞ A Study-Supplement to Kent's Lectures on Materia Medica, 2nd Edition

CONTENTS

CONTENTS

1. WORDS OF INSPIRATION

WIDE STUDY

"One consults and **quotes from several of our prescribing** geniuses **because,** one man has more completely grasped the inwardness and has had more experience with one remedy, another with another. For the same reason, it is well to read and study the **same drug in several books** to get enlightment always from the man who is best qualified to enlighten. **Pick plenty of brains if you want to nourish and stimulate your own.**"

Dr. M.L. Tyler

OPEN MIND

"Homeopathy, if properly understood, **offers** a distinct contribution to medicine, and it has been a narrow conception of what constitutes the healing art that has excluded it from the general profession. That of itself it has fallen into the **hands of the incompetent and unscrupulous is no excuse for failing to investigate its actual merits. If the science of medicine is to be restricted to its own discoveries it is doomed.**"

Dr. C.M. Boger

NEED OF HIGH GRADE LITERATURE

"We not only need, but must have homeopathic literature of a higher grade to interpret our art in an **appealing, intelligent, concise,** and **convincing** manner to the intelligent mind.

Dr. Arthur B. Green

DIET

"The physician who fails to correct and **simplify the diet** in harmony with good sense is unintentionally having serious obstacles to recovery unremoved and to that extent he is falling short of the physician's highest and the only calling which is to *restore health to the sick."*

Dr. Underhill

DR. NASH OBSERVES

It is curious to note that almost every **chemical** remedy has a closely resembling relative from **vegetable** kingdom. Phytolacca and Kali hydriodicum, Aloes and Sulphur, Cepa and Phosphorus, Chamomilla and Magnesia carb., China and Ferrum, Belladonna and Calcarea ost., Ipecac. and Cuprum, Bryonia and Alumina, Mezerium and Mercury, Pulsatilla and Kali sulph.

This has been before mentioned by **Hering.**

This **Phenomenon** of the Homeopathic world has been especially highlighted by Dr. J.T. Kent.

(Quoted from "Two Stars of Homeopathy" by the Author)

---

2. WONDERS OF A SINGLE DOSE

ALOE SOC.: (Constipation) I was called to treat a **child** five years of age **suffering** from birth with a most **obstinate form of constipation.** He had to be forced and held to the stool, crying and screaming all the while, being totally unable to pass any faeces even after an enema. I then gave a few doses of *Aloe 200th* and cured the whole trouble quickly and **permanently.**

Dr. E.B. Nash

ANTIMONIUM TART.—(Vomit) it has the nausea, vomiting, loose stools, prostration, cold sweat, and stupor or drowsiness found in almost all bad cases of this disease, and **I have seldom** been obliged to give **more than two or three doses,** one after each vomiting before the case was relieved.

Dr. E.B. Nash

ARNICA MONT.: (Parturition) I have come to the conclusion that in every case after the **delivery,** absolutely in every case, **I have to give a dose of** *Arnica,* I have never had the slightest trouble in many cases, because I always have Arnica, and in **abortions,** after the abortion, always *Arnica,* and there is always something more to come, and it comes out easily and everything is safe, and **absolutely no lesion.**

Dr. F.K. Bellokossy

ARNICA: (Sprain) I have seen a **sprained ankle** when it was black and blue, so swollen that the shoe could not be put on, but after a dose of *Arnica*, the swelling disappeared in an astonishing way, the discolouration faded out and the patient was able to stand on the foot.

Dr.J.T.Kent

ARSENICUM ALB.: (sciatica) one of the worst cases of sciatica I ever saw was cured with *Arsenicum album*, on the indications, worse at midnight, especially from 1 to 3 o'clock; burning pains; and the only temporary relief during the paroxysms, was from bags of hot, dry salt applied to the painful part.

The lady was a sister of Charles Saunders, of New York, of school reader fame, who was himself a **cripple** from allopathically treated sciatica. She, after suffering indescribable agony for six weeks, was cured **rapidly and permanently** with a dose of Jenichen's 8m. of *Arsenicum album*. So we see again that no remedy and **no particular set of remedies can be entirely relied upon, but the indicated one can.**

Dr.E.B. Nash

ARSENICUM ALB.: (Asthma) I remember a case of asthma of long standing duration to which I was called at midnight, because they were afraid that the patient would die before morning. Found that her attacks always come on at 1 A.M. Gave *Arsenicum alb*.30th, and she was completely cured by it.

Dr. E.B. Nash

AURUM MUR NAT.: (Liver Troubles) While on a visit to New York City, I called upon Dr.M.Baruch, partly to see the man who had been reported to me as both, very **skillful** as a prescriber and **eccentric** as a man. During my call I stated to him my case. He prescribed for me a dose of *Aurum muriaticum natronatum* 1000th, followed by a powder each of *veronica officinalis* 500th, 200th and 30th, and directed me to take them in the order named **once in sixty hours and said:** "In **three months you will be well.**" I took the powders as directed and have never been troubled in that way since.

Dr. E.B.Nash

BELLADONNA: (Breast) The elder Lippe once told me of a case of suspicious enlargement or swelling and pain of the **breast** of long standing, which, as he expressed it, seemed likely to prove a case for the surgeon (cancer), which was entirely cured by a few doses of *Belladonna*, to which he was guided by this symptom of the pains being so much **worse on lying down.** Since then I have observed and verified this symptom in many cases of different kinds.

Dr. E.B. Nash

CADMIUM: (Cancer of liver) I frequently find cancer of the liver yielding to *Calcarea ars.* in every way but with the **tendency to relapse, when a single dose of cadmium in high potency will render the cure permanent.**

Dr. A.H. Grimmer

CALCAREA-CARB: (Lime assimilation) It is astonishing that one single dose of the potency suitable, to meet the state of disorder will make that **infant** commence to **digest its food,** and **appropriate** from its food the lime substance that it needs in its bones, and wherever else it needs it. All at once the **teeth** begin to grow; the bones begin to grow; and the **legs get stiff** enough for him to begin to walk; and they will hold him up. **It is astonishing** what changes will take place under the various medicines that are suitable for the disturbances of the **hair,** the **bones** and the **nails.**

Dr. J.T. Kent

CAUSTICUM: (Suppressed eczema) I was once called, in consultation, to a case of **prosopalgia** which had for a long time baffled the skill of a very good homeopathic practitioner. Not being able to relieve the case, he had become demoralized, and as the pain and suffering were very great he had resorted to anodynes, but with the usual result of making the patient worse, (after the anodynes had worn out), than she was before. On looking over the case carefully, I found in addition to the emaciated and greatly **debilitated** condition of the patient, after so long suffering, that the pains came in **paroxysms,** that they were **of a drawing nature,** and that she had suffered from **eczema for years,** at different times, before this pain appeared. *Sulphur* had been given, but without relief. So I advised *Causticum.* It was given, in the 200th, and a rapid and a permanent cure was the result.

Dr. E.B. Nash

CHAMOMILLA: (Irritation) **Dr. Tyrell** said once to me: "when the **husband** complains of the **wife's** being **cross** and **irritable** and he cannot get along with her, give him a dose of *Chamomilla* and it has worked. I have done it many times.

Dr. Edwards

CHINA OFF.: (Bleeding) After profuse bleeding in delivery, a dose of china 1M, dilution will **recoup the strength** of the patient.

Dr. R.B. Das

COLCHICUM AUT.: (Bloody stools) The **smell of cooking food nauseates** to faintness. To illustrate the value of this symptom I will give a case of my own practice; it was also my first experience with a potency as high as the 200th. Patient was a lady, seventy-five years of age, who was suddenly seized with sickness at the stomach and vomiting of blood in large quantities; then bloody stools followed, which were at first profuse, then became small and of bloody mucus. There was great tenesmus and pain in the bowels. She had become so weak that she could not lift her head from the pillow. By actual count the number of **stools** passed on clothes in the bed **was sixty-five, in twenty-four hours,** the pains, number of passages and all symptoms were **aggravated from sundown to sunrise.** One dose in above potency cured her.

Dr. E.B. Nash

GRAPHITES: (Scar) If you know a woman who is suffering from an **old scar** that has formed a lump, when she is about to go into confinement, give a dose of *Graphites* as a general **remedy, unless some other special remedy is called for.**

Dr. J.T. Kent

GRAPHITES: (Eczema) I once treated a case of **eczema** of the **legs** which was of twenty years standing. It was in an old **obese** woman, and, by the way, that is the kind of subject in which this remedy is found most efficacious.

I gave her, on account of much **burning of the feet,** a dose of *Sulphur* cm. In two or three weeks an eruption was developed all over the body which exuded a glutinous sticky fluid. One dose of *Graphites* cm., dry on the tongue, cured this as well as the eczema of the legs and left her skin as smooth as that of a child.

Dr.E.B. Nash

GRAPHITES: (Suppressed eczema) A child three years of age had eczema capitis. **Under allopathic local treatment,** the eczema disappeared; but soon entero-colitis of a very obstinate character set in. Then the regulars could not "do" that as they had the eczema, and after they had given up the case, pronouncing it consumption of the bowels, the homeopath (myself) was called in on the ground that he could do no harm if he could do no good (as they said).

Case: Child greatly emaciated, little or no appetite, very restless, and "stools brown fluid mixed with undigested substances, and of an intolerably foetid odor." taking into the account the history of the suppressed eczema I prescribed *Graphites* 6m. (Jenichen) and in a short **time a perfect cure was the result.**

Dr. E.B. Nash

HEDERA HELIX: (Hydrocephalus - Blocked nose) Given **Hedera helix one drop one dose** only. Next morning clear flow of fluid through the nose will appear and only one dose will cure. Give second dose if recurrence is threatened.

IODIUM: (goitre) I have cured many cases of goitre with *Iodine* cm., every night for four nights, after the moon fulled and was waning.

Dr. E.B. Nash

IRIS VERS.: (Vomit) I once had a case of stomach trouble in a middle-aged lady. She had frequent attacks of vomiting of a stringy, glairy mucus which was very ropy, would hang in strings from her mouth to the receptacle on the floor. Then the substance vomited became dark-coloured; like coffee grounds. She became very weak, vomited all nourishment. She also had profuse secretion of ropy saliva.

Thinking she had cancer of the stomach, she made her will and set her house in order, to die. *Kali bich.* was given with no benefit whatever, but *Iris vers.* **cured her completely** in a short time and she remains well ten years since.

Dr. E.B. Nash

KALIUM CARB. : (Dropsy) The father-in-law of Dr. T.L. Brown, an anaemic old man, was apparently near his end with hydrothorax and general dropsy. Dr. Brown was a skillful prescriber, but in this case had utterly failed to even relieve. In consultation with Dr. Sioan, after carefully reviewing the case, the fact appeared through the daughter of the patient, who had been his nurse all the time, that all his symptoms were **aggravated at 3 A.M.** Now *Kali carb.* 200 was given, and with such miraculous results that in an incredibly short time the old man was well and never had a return of that trouble. **He lived for several years** after, and, finally, did not die of dropsy at all.

Dr. E.B. Nash

KALIUM IOD.: (Hives) **A single dose of a very high potency** of *Kali iod.* will turn things into order in persons subject to these **hives** and they will not come again.

Dr. J.T. Kent

LACHESIS: (Long action) In many cases, the action of one dose not only lasts for several days, weeks and months but sometimes **one or two doses of Lachesis** have cured the very chronic and the most complicated cases for ever

Dr. B. Prasad Gupta

LACHESIS: (Headache) Headache extending into nose, comes mostly in acute catarrh, especially when the discharge has been suppressed or stops after sleep. This kind of headache is often found in hay fever, with frequent and violent paroxysms of sneezing. Now, if the hay fever paroxysms of a sneezing are decidedly **worse after sleeping, even in the day time,** Lachesis 200th may stop the whole business for the season.

Dr. E.B. Nash

LACHESIS: (Colic) I once had a case of very obstinate constipation in an old syphilitic case. He was at last taken with very severe attacks of colic. The pains seemed to extend all through the abdomen, and always came on **at night.** After trying various remedies until I was discouraged, for he "got no better fast," he let drop this expression, **"Doctor, if I could only keep awake all the time, I would never have another attack."** I looked askance at him. "I mean," said he, "that I sleep into the attack, and waken in it." I left a dose of *Lachesis* 200. He never had another attack of the pain, and his bowels became perfectly regular from that day and remained so.

Dr. E.B. Nash

LACHESIS: (Dyspnoea) In chronic cases wait patiently and see its deep and intense action. I have seen its working of **one dose of thirty potency for months.** One dose of thirty dilution has cured in my hands not only one case but patients after patients. In one case, dyspnoea with heart palpitation, severe and intolerable pains of left side before menses, blackish menses, falling of hair, over-sensitive to light etc., all these **symptoms were of several years** and one dose of thirty potency cured.

Dr. B. Prasad Gupta

LYCOPODIUM: (Impotence) It is one of our best remedies for impotence. An old man marries his second or third wife and finds himself not "equal to the occasion." it is very embarrassing for the whole family. **A dose of** *Lycopodium* **sets** the thing all right and makes the doctor a warm friend on both sides of the house.

Young men from onanism or sexual excess become impotent. The penis becomes small, cold and relaxed. The desire is as strong as ever, and perhaps more so, but he can't perform. (*Selenium, Caladium*). I have known apparently hopeless cases of this kind cured by the use of this remedy, high single doses at intervals of a week or more. Give it low, however, if you want to, but do not blame me if you don't succeed.

Dr. E.B. Nash

MAGNESIA-CARB: (Coccydynia) I once cured a severe case of Coccydynia, a case of long standing. The pains were sudden, piercing, causing the patient to almost faint away. Magnesia carb. 200 cured promptly.

Dr. E.B. Nash

MERCURIUS SOL.: (Coryza) The chill is peculiar as I have observed it. It is not a shaking chill, but is simply **creeping chilliness.** Often when this creeping chilliness is felt, it is the first symptom of a cold that has been taken, and, if left alone, the coryza, sore throat, bronchitis or even pneumonia may follow; but, if taken early, a dose of *Mercurius* may prevent all such troubles. The chilliness is felt most generally in the **evening** and **increases during the night,** if not removed by mercury. It also alternates with flashes of heat; first chilly, then hot, then chilly, etc., like *Arsenicum alb.* It is often felt in **single parts.** Then again it is felt in abscesses and is the **harbinger of pus formation.** If pus has already formed, especially much of it, the only thing *Mercury* can do is to hasten its discharge; but if little or none is actually formed, a dose of Mercury high potency will often check the formation and **a profuse sweat often follows** with a subsidence of the swelling and a rapid cure of the disease.

Dr. E.B. Nash

MERCURIUS SOL.: (High potency) If anyone is skeptical as to the **efficiency of the very high potencies,** I invite him to a test in just such a case. Give a single dose, dry upon the tongue or if you must seem to do more, dissolve a powder in four tablespoonfuls of water and **give in half-hourly doses.** Then wait, I have done it many times and am convinced.

Dr. E.B. Nash

NATRIUM MUR.: (Loss of weight) I have seen a patient who had lost 40 pounds of flesh (weight, 160 1b.), though eating well all of the time, under **one dose of** Natrum mur., tip the scales at 200 1bs. within three months from the time of taking, he was very **hypochondriac** at the time of the beginning of treatment.

Dr. E.B. Nash

NUX VOMICA: (Peristalsis) Inefficient labour pains, extending to rectum, with desire for stool or frequent urination, are quickly relieved, and become efficient, after the administration of a dose of *Nux vomica* 200.

Dr. E.B. Nash

PETROLEUM: (Eczema) I have cured a case of eczema of the lower legs of **twenty years standing,** always worse in winter, with one prescription of *Petroleum* 200th. I have cured chapped hands the same way. I once had a very obstinate case of chronic diarrhea, but as soon as the fact that he had **eczema of the hands in winter** came to light I cured him quickly of the whole trouble with petroleum 200.

Dr. E.B. Nash

PLUMBUM MET.: (Paralysis) I cured one case of post diphtheritic paralysis with it. It was a very severe case in a middle-aged man. His lower limbs were entirely paralyzed, and there was at the same time a symptom which I never met before, nor have I since, in such a case, viz., **excessive hyperaesthesia of the skin.** He could **not bear to be touched** anywhere, it hurt him so. After much hunting I found this hyperaesthesia perfectly pictured in Allen's Encyclopaedia, and that, taken **together with the paralysis,** seemed to me good reason for prescribing *Plumbum met.,* which I did in one dose of Fincke's 40m., with the result of bringing about rapid and continuous improvement until a perfect cure was reached. He **took only the one dose,** for a repetition was not necessary.

Dr. E.B. Nash

PLUMBUM MET.: (Typhlitis) The father-in-law of Dr. T.L.Brown, over seventy years of age, was attacked with a severe pain in the abdomen. Finally, a large, hard swelling developed in the ileo-caecal region very sensitive to contact or to the least motion. It began to assume a bluish colour, and on account of his age and extreme weakness, it was thought that he must die. His daughter, however, studied up the case, and found in Raue's pathology the indications for *Plumbum met* as given in therapeutic hints for **typhlitis**. It was administered in the *200th potency*, which was followed by relief and perfect recovery.

Dr. E.B. Nash

PSORINUM: (Skin) It is also found useful in the consequences of suppressed eruptions, and in such cases should never be forgotten when other anti-psorics fail. Dr. Wm. A. Hawley, of Syracuse, N.Y., once made a brilliant cure of a very **bad case of dropsy** in an old woman, being led to prescribe this remedy by the appearance of the skin. One dose of Fincke's 42m. potency, dry on the tongue, cured the whole case in a very short time.

Dr. E.B. Nash

SILICEA: (Epilepsy) I have several times found a Silicea child suffering from epileptiform spasms which were always **worse at new moon.** A few doses of *Silicea* 200 set them all right.

Dr. E.B. Nash

STAPHYSAGRIA: (Warts) In one case, with the 200th potency of this remedy, I removed an excrescence on the perineum of a lady in which the growth was an inch long and the appearance was exactly like cauliflower. It rapidly disappeared under the action of this remedy and never returned.

Dr. E.B. Nash

STICTA PULMONARIA: (Insomnia) When after a wound, sprain or fracture, the patient tells you, "Since my accident, I do not have sound sleep; I sleep badly; one dose of *Sticta pulmonaria* 200 brings sleep. This is a remedy with the characteristic that it **does not habitually** work on insomnia, but it makes the **fracture victim sleep.**

Dr. Pierre Schmidt

SYPHILINUM: (Asthma) It has cured spasmodic bronchial asthma of twenty-five years standing.

Dr. B. Prasad Gupta

TUBERCULINUM: (Headache) Dr. Swan cured a case of headache of forty-five years standing with Tuberculinum.

Dr. B. Prasad Gupta

TUBERCULINUM: (Retarted menses) One case of **retarded menstruation** in a young girl who had greatly enlarged tonsils and who began to grow tired and weak, pale and short breathed on any exercise. The menses appeared twice under the action of *Pulsatilla*, but at intervals of several months, and finally not at all. After the failure of several other remedies to give her any benefit, she took one dose of *Tuberculinum* 1M. with prompt, easy and natural appearance of the menses and corresponding improvement in other respects, and is now attending school in apparent good health.

Dr. E.B. Nash

TUBERCULINUM: (Lung trouble) A case of lung trouble brought to me over a year ago from Seneca falls, N.Y., had been under allopathic treatment for four years and had been in every summer up in the Adirondacks at Saranac, at a sanitarium established by Dr. Loomis, of New York, lung specialist. She continued to grow worse until I took her case in hand. Under the action of 2 doses of *Sulphur* cm. followed by *Tuberculinum* cm. she is so improved that I think it would be hard to convince any one that she ever suffered from such conditions.

Dr. E.B. Nash

HOMEOPATHY GETTING RELIGIOUS IN ITS ATTITUDE

Originally and basically religion is a science, a science of spirit and its realization. But in course of time, the phenomenon has changed. It has gained unlimited forms and **conceptions.** "Hari Anant Hari Katha Ananta" God is beyond limit, and the ways to find them are unlimited.

Homeopathy was in its origin, a **pure science.** Hahnemann wanted to make it a **mathematical science** in certainty. But in course of time, the 'pathy' adopted 'Art' and 'Religion' for its 'form.'

As in religion, everybody own's a God of his on own, so in homeopathy, everybody has his own 'pathy' and form - whatever it may be.

(Quoted from "The reality" by the author)

3. 'SHEET ANCHOR' IN EMERGENCIES

ARNICA TINCTURE: Applied neat to a **wasp** or **bee sting** is wonderfully effective.

Dr. M.Blackey

CALCAREA CARB.: When given in repeated dose of 30th dilution relieves the pain attending the **biliary passage.**

Dr. Hughes

COLOCYNTHIS: No remedy produces more **severe colic** than this one, and no remedy cures more promptly.

Dr. E.B. Nash

HYPERICUM PERF.: Quite supercedes the use of morphia **after operations** in my hand.

Dr. Helmuth

Nothing equals Hypericum in cases of **mashed fingers.**

Dr. E.A. Farrington

MURIATICUM ACID: Is useful in the last stage of **dropsy** from Cirrhosis of liver.

Dr. E.A. Farrington

MYRISTICA SEB. 3x: Called the **homeopathic knife**, is almost specific drug to **break open Carbuncle.**

Dr. W. Karo

MYRISTICA SEB.: Often does away with the use of knife. Acts more powerfully than any other remedy **in carbuncle**.

Dr. C.C. Boericke

NATRUM MUR.: Is one of our best remedies for **chronic headaches**.

Dr. E.B. Nash

SPIGELIA: In the few cases of **pericarditis,** I have treated, *spigelia* has done all that medicine could do.

Dr. Russell

STRAMONIUM: Is most important when **pain is almost unbearable,** driving to despair. It ameliorates at once, and hastens benign suppuration.

Dr. C.G. Raue

SYMPHYTUM OFF.: Fracture of hand and finger bones: these knit more quickly with *Symphytum* 30 two or three times a day for a week.

Dr. Pierre Schmidt

4. QUICKEST PALLIATION POSSIBLE

ACONITUM NAP.: If **dysentery** sets in with violent fever, *Aconite* in many cases cures the whole disease in 2 or 3 days.

Dr. Jahr

ANTIMONIUM CRUD.: It is especially to be considered if the **gastric derangement** is of **recent date.** The process of digestion is hardly under way; the eructations taste of the food as he ate it, and the sufferer feels as if he must **"throw up"** before there will be any relief. In such a case a few pellets of *Antimonium crudum* on the tongue will often settle the business, **save the loss of a meal,** and all further suffering.

Dr. E.B. Nash

ANTIMONIUM SULPH. NIG.: it relieves **itching** of skin which frequently occurs in **old people.**

Dr. Rudolph F. Rabe

ARNICA MONT.: If given at once after a fracture, it almost instantly relieves the **muscular spasms** which often occur and also relieves the shock.

Dr. Stearns

ARNICA MONT.: Given immediately **in fractures** and dislocations, relieves the nervousness and pain like magic, both externally and internally.

Dr. R. Patel & Dr. Elias

ARNICA will quiet the startlings of a fractured limb.

Dr. Hughes

ARNICA MONT.: It is very beneficial not only in injuries caused by severe contusions and lacerations of fibres, but also in the most **severe wounds by bullets and blunt weapons;** in the pains and other ailments consequent on extracting the teeth and other surgical operations whereby sensitive parts have been violently stretched; as also after dislocations of joints, after setting fractures of bones etc.

Dr. Samuel Hahnemann

CALCAREA SULPH.: I once had a case in which there was great pain in the region of the kidneys for a day and night. Then there was a great discharge of **pus in the urine,** which continued several days and weakened the patient very fast. A Chicago specialist had examined the urine a short time before, and had pronounced the case as **Bright's disease.** I finally prescribed *Cacarea sulphurica* 12 and under its action she immediately improved and made a very rapid and permanent recovery.

Dr. E.B. Nash

CANTHARIS VES.: *Cantharis* 200 given internally, quickly cures the inflamed and horrible swelling that may follow **gnat bites.**

Dr. M.L. Tyler

CAUSTICUM: In 6th dilution will give immediate relief to pain in cases of **burns and scalds.**

Dr. R.B. Das

CAUSTICUM: It is the routine remedy for **retention of urine** after operation.

Dr. D.M. Foubister

CHAMOMILLA: It will stop **vomiting of morphia** in a few minutes.

Dr. J.K. Kent

CHOLESTERINUM: It is specific for **gall stone colic;** relieves the distress at once.

Dr. Swan

CINA MAR.: I once had, at one time, and in one family, five cases of **typhoid fever,** and they were all very sick. There was no mistake about the diagnosis, and I speak this positively, because some think that a child under the age of six years cannot have this disease. **This child, five years of age,** was the last one of the family attacked with the disease, and it pursued the same course as the others in its regular rise and fall of temperature, bloating of abdomen, diarrhea and other symptoms common to this disease. I resolved to give **a few doses of** *Cina* anyway, and to my surprise I found my patient much better in every way at my next visit and the improvement progressed right along to complete recovery. I learned for good, that, for purposes of prescribing, the **name of the disease** was of little account.

Dr. E.B. Nash

COLOCYNTHIS: If I was disposed to be skeptical as to the power of the small dose to cure, *Colocynthis* would convince me, for I have so promptly **cured severe colic** in many cases, from a child to adults, and even in horses. Of course, every true homeopath can respond a man to that.

DIGITALIS PUR. : One day I saw an old but very strong man staggering across the road towards my office. I thought he was drunk, but on close observation I noticed that his face looked purple, his lips bluish, and I stepped out and helped him in. He sat down and could not speak a word, for a few minutes and **struggled for breath.** His pulse was very irregular and intermittent. He had been obliged to give up all manual labour and dared not go away from home on his business, that of bridge builder. He expected to die with his heart disease. **I gave him** *Digitalis* **2,** a few drops in water. In a few days I saw him shoveling snow from the walk in front of his dwelling. "Hello," he said, "I have no heart disease;" and I saw him often after that and he told me that the medicine cured him of "those spells."

Dr. E.B. Nash

HAMAMELIS VIR.: In **varicose veins** of the leg, you will be delighted with the way in which the first or second dilution of Hamamelis will cure the pain.

Dr. Hughes

HYOSCYAMUS NIG.: It is is one of our best remedies for **hiccough** occurring after **operations** of the abdomen.

Dr. E.A. Farrington

LAPIS ALB.: I put her upon *Lapis album* as an experiment, for I had no hope she could live more than two weeks at the longest. Under the action of this remedy she began to improve immediately, and from the half dead wreck that could not turn in bed without help, a skeleton, white as a ghost, she has steadily improved until she is now doing her own housework, the discharges having all ceased except her natural menses at her regular periods. **The tumor grows**

smaller, and it seems as though she might get well. She takes a dose of *Lapis album* 30th once a week.

Dr. E.B. Nash

PICRICUM AC.: I found this remedy very useful in apparent failure of **brain power** in an old man who had always been strong up to within a year or so of the time he called on me. He complained of heaviness in the occiput and **inability to exert the mind to talk or think,** and general tired **"played-out" feeling.** I feared brain softening but I gave him *Picric acid* 6th trit. and it promptly cured him.

Dr. E.B. Nash

PLANTAGO MIN.: Toothache with the 2x dilution of *Plantago,* I cure seven-tenths of all cases of this kind in about 15 minutes.

Dr. Ruetlinger

PULSATILLA: *Pulsatilla* will very often cause in five minutes a very strong **contraction of the uterus,** sometimes almost in a painless way.

Dr. J.T. Kent

RHUS TOX: It is the homeopathic knife in **appendicitis.**

Dr. Biegler

RHUS TOX is beneficial to control the **threatened Iritis and formation of pus.**

Dr. Dewey

SECALE COR.: All the toes were attacked with **dry gangrene.** A few doses of Secale(high potency) afforded great relief, and checked the progress of the disease for a long time.

Dr. E.B. Nash

STAPHYSAGRIA: It is required when an abdominal or other **operation wound is unduly painful** for no obvious reason.

Dr. D.M. Foubister

TARENTULA CUB.: I have seen **felons** which had kept patients awake night after night, walking the floor in agony from the **terrible pains,** so relieved in a very short time that they could sleep in perfect comfort until the swellings spontaneously discharged, and progressed to a rapid cure.

Dr. E.B. Nash

THUJA OCC.: A case of **enuresis** had resisted many seemingly indicated remedies, until the hands were discovered to be covered with **warts,** when a few drops of *Thuja* cured.

Dr. E.B. Nash

VIBERNUM OP. Q: Cramps in the abdomen and **legs of pregnant** women are controlled very quickly by this remedy.

Dr. Hale

5. MIRACULUS CURES IN DIFFICULT, CHRONIC AND INCURABLE DISEASES

AMMONIUM CARB.: It has **cured the cough of influenza** when every thing else has failed, and I have not found it necessary to give a second dose IN MANY CASES.

Dr. Younan

ANACARDIUM ORI.: In the fall of 1899 I was called to a lady, married, 35 years of age, mother of three children.

She was quite emaciated, with a yellowish cachectic look of the face. A couple of years before I treated her when she had an attack **of vomiting,** in which she vomited coffee ground substances.

She was relieved at that time by a dose of *Arsenicum alb.* 40m., but had more or less trouble with her digestion up to this time. This last attack was more persistent and did not yield to *Arsenicum* and some other remedies.

After a while it appeared that the pain (which was very severe) and **vomiting came on when the stomach was empty.** She had to eat once or twice in the night for relief. The substance vomited was always black or brown looking like

coffee-grounds. Her sister had been operated for cancer of
the breast, and of course she was very nervous and fearful
of cancer of the stomach, *Anacardium* relieved promptly, and
she has had no return of the trouble since then.

Dr. E.B. Nash

ANTIMONIUM CRUD.: There is a **form of diarrhea
which alternates with constipation,** oftenest found with old
people, where *Antimonium crudum* is the only remedy. then
it is also one of the best remedies for mucus piles; there is a
continuous oozing of mucus staining the linen, very
disagreeable to the patient.

Dr. E.B. Nash

ANTIMONIUM CRUD.: Some of the worst cases of
chronic rheumatism have been cured by this remedy, guided
by the excessive **tenderness of the soles of the feet.**

Dr. E.B. Nash

APIS MEL.: Sensation as if **every breath would be his
last,** is very characteristic, and occurs not only in dropsical
troubles of the chest, but seems also to be a **nervous
symptom.**

Dr. E.B. Nash

APIS MEL.: a number of years ago, I was called to
Watkins glen, N.Y., for consultation in a very bad case of
diphtheria. One had already died in the family and four lay
dead in the place that day. **Over forty cases had died** in the
place and there was an exodus going on for fair. Her
attending physician, a noble, white-haired old man, and a
good and able man, said, when I looked up to him and
remarked, I was rather young to counsel him; "Doctor, I am

on my knees to anybody, for every case has died that has been attacked." The patient was two rooms away from us, but I could hear her **difficult breathing even then.** *Apis* was comparatively a new remedy then for that disease, but as I looked into her throat I saw *Apis* in a moment, and a few questions confirmed it. I told the doctor what I thought and asked him if he had tried it. He said, no, **he had not thought of it,** but it was a powerful blood poison; try it. It cured the case, and **not one case** that took this remedy from the beginning, and persistently, died. **It was the remedy for the genus epidemicus.**

Dr. E.B. Nash

ARGENTUM MET.: You will be astonished to know that homeopathic remedies are wonderful in their ability to create tonicity, and thereby restore the **prolapsed uterus to its normal position,** and to remove the dragging down feeling women generally describe, a sensation as if the inner parts were being forced out. *Argentum met.* **is one of them.**

Dr. J.T. Kent

ARGENTUM NIT.: It has cured prolonged and most inveterate **ulceration of the stomach,** when there has been vomiting of blood.

Dr. J.T. Kent

ARGENTUM NIT.: In dull **chronic headaches** of literary and businessman, *Argentum nitricum* is most commended.

Dr. Hughes

ARNICA MONT.: I have come to the conclusion that in every case after the **delivery,** absolutely in every case, I have to give a dose of *Arnica,* I have never had the slightest trouble in many cases, because I always have Arnica, and **in abortions,** after the abortion, always *Arnica,* and there is always something more to come, and it comes out easily and everything is safe, and absolutely no lesion.

Dr. F.K. Bellocossy

ARNICA MONT.: I once cured a man who had suffered from what he and his physician had called **dyspepsia** for several years. He had been obliged to give up his business because he could not eat enough to support his strength. He had been told by his physician that he would never be well again and had given up hopes himself. This condition was caused by the **kick of a horse upon the region of the stomach.** A few doses of *Arnica* 200 cured him in a short time and he resumed his business.

Dr. E.B. Nash

BORAX VEN.: The ears discharge. I cured a case of otorrhea of fourteen years standing with this remedy.

Dr. E.B. Nash

CANTHARIS: The mucus was so profuse, and tenacious, and ropy, that I thought of *Kali bichromicum,* and thought it must be the remedy; **but it did not even ameliorate,** and she got worse all the time, until one day she mentioned that she had great **cutting and burning on** urinating, which she must do very frequently.

On the strength of the urinary symptom, for I knew nothing of its **curative powers on the respiratory organs** at that time, I gave her *Cantharis.* The effect was magical.

It is needless to describe the mutual delight of both physician and patient in such a case, for it was so astonishing rapidity with which the perfect and permanent cure of the case was accomplished.

Dr. E.B. Nash

CANNABIS SAT.: It is the remedy par excellence with which to begin the **treatment of gonorrhoea,** unless some other remedy is particularly indicated, and such cases are very few. The most characteristic symptom is that the **urethra is very sensitive to touch** or external pressure. The patient **cannot walk with his legs close together** because any pressure along the tract hurts him so. If the diseases has extended up the urethra, or into the bladder, there will often be severe **pains in the back** every few minutes and the **urine may be bloody.** I, in my early practice, used to put five drops mother tincture into four ounces of water (in a four-ounce vial) and let the patient take a teaspoonful three times a day. After about four days, the inflammatory symptoms would have subsided, and the thin discharge have thickened and become greenish in appearance. **Then** *Mercurius solubilis* **3rd** trituration, a powder three times a day, would often finish the case. **If a little, thin, gleety discharge remained,** I cured that with *Sulphur, Capsicum* or *Kali iodide*. I have cured many cases from one to two weeks this way. **Later I have used the c.m. potency in the first stage,** and sometimes never have to use the **second remedy.** If I do, *Mercurius* C.M. is generally the remedy. **Sometimes** *Pulsatilla, Sulphur,* or *Sepia* to finish up the case. There are exceptions, but the rule is that the cases get well promptly under this treatment.

Dr. E.B. Nash

CARBO AN.: It has temporarily relieved in incurable cases and has apparently removed the cancerous condition for years, even though it comes back afterwards and kills.

This remedy is often a great **palliative** for the **pains that occur in cancer,** the indurations and the stinging, burning pains.

Of course we do not want to teach, nor we wish to have you infer, that a patient with a well-advanced cancerous affection, such as scirrhus, may, be restored to perfect health, and the cancerous affection removed.

Any one who goes around boasting of the cancer cases he has cured, ought to be regarded with suspicion.

Dr. J.T. Kent

CARBO VEG.: Vital force nearly exhausted, cold surface, especially from knees down to feet; lies motionless, as if dead; breath cold; pulse intermittent, thready; cold sweat on limbs. This is truly a desperate condition. Then add to these symptoms, **blood stagnates in the capillaries,** causing blueness, coldness and ecchymoses; the patient so weak that he cannot breathe without being constantly fanned. Gasps: " fan me: fan me:" Carbo veg. has saved such cases.

Dr. E.B. Nash

CARBO VEG.: Chronic complaints following or dating back for years to some **imperfectly cured** or **suppressed acute disease.**

Dr. E.B. Nash

CAUSTICUM: This is like *Nux vomica* and *Cantharis,* and I once cured a chronic case of **cystitis** in a married woman, which had baffled the best efforts of several old school physicians, eminent for their skill, for years.

Dr. E.B. Nash

CHINA OFF.: It is one of the best remedies in **chronic liver troubles.** There is pain in the right hypochondria, and often the liver may be felt below the ribs, enlarged, hard and **sensitive to touch.**

Dr. E.B. Nash

CISTUS CAN.: I remember the first time my attention was decidedly called to *Cistus.* I had put it on my list to study from that time and have come to the conclusion that it was only a side issue, until a young lady, nineteen years of age fell under my observation. The **glands of the neck** were enlarged and hard, the parotids especially. She had foetid **otorrhoea;** her eyes were inflamed and suppurating; there were fissures at the corners of the eyes; her **lips were cracked** and bleeding, and she had **salt rheum at the end of the fingers.** I could not make *Calcarea* fit to the patient but after much study this little remedy seemed to be just what I needed; and **although she had an immense amount of homeopathy, good and bad, this remedy cured.**

Dr. J.T.Kent

COLLINSONIA CAN.: With Collinsonia I once cured a very **severe colic** which had been of frequent occurrence in a lady for several years and had completely baffled the old school efforts to cure. I was led to choose the remedy on account of the **obstinate constipation,** the great flatulence and the hemorrhoidal condition present.

Dr. E.B. Nash

CONIUM MAC.: It is perhaps the first remedy to be thought of in all cases of **tumors,** scirrhous or otherwise, coming on after contusions, especially if they are of **stony hardness** and heavy feeling.

Dr. E.B. Nash

CROTALUS HOR.: It seems, so far, to have shown its greatest usefulness in diseases which result in a **decomposition of the blood** of such a character as to cause haemorrhages from **every outlet of the body** (*Acetic acid*); **even the sweat is bloody.**

Dr. E.B. Nash

CHELIDONIUM MAJ.: Sometimes in **coughs which are persistent with much pain through right side of the chest** and into the shoulder, *Chelidonium* **helps us out** and saves the patient from what might easily terminate in **consumption.**

Dr. E.B. Nash

COLCHICUM AUT.: I had my Lippe's text-book of Materia Medica in my carriage. I went out, got it and sat down by the bedside; determined to find that peculiar and persistent symptom and "fight it out on that line if it took all summer." I had a box of Dunham's 200ths under my carriage seat that had been there for over a year, but which I have never used for **want of confidence in high potencies.** It was the best I could do for the present, so I dissolved a few pellets in a half glass of cold water, and directed to give one teaspoonful after every passage of the bowels. On my way home, I stopped my horse two or three times to turn around and go back and give that poor suffering woman some medicine. I felt guilty, but I said to myself, **"this is Lippe's Materia Medica,** and these are **Carrol Dunham's potencies,** and here is a clear cut indication for its administration, and the other symptoms do not counter-indicate." Well, I got home. But I started early the next morning to try and make amends for my rashness (if the patient was not dead) of yesterday. Imagine my surprise as I stepped into the sick-room when my patient slowly turned her head upon the pillow and said, with a smile, "good morning, doctor." I had been met with a groan several past mornings. I felt faint myself then. I dropped into a chair by the bedside and remarked, "you are feeling better?" "Oh, yes, doctor." "How much of that last medicine did you take?" **"Two doses."** "What!" "Two doses"; **"I only had two more stools after you left."** "Don't you have any more pain?" **"Pain stopped like that"** (putting her hands together) "and I feel well except weakness." She took no more medicine, quickly recovered, and was perfectly well for five years after.

Dr. E.B. Nash

HELLEBORUS NIG.: These symptoms, **head rolling from side to side on the pillow,** with screams; great stupidity or soporous sleep; **greedy drinking of water;** wrinkled forehead with cold sweat; motion of jaws, as chewing something; **continual motion of one arm and leg,** while the other lies as if paralyzed; urine scanty or **entirely suppressed,** (sometimes sediment like coffee grounds) indicated a desperate condition, and the patient will soon die, comatose or in convulsions unless the proper remedy can be found.

Helleborus niger can often cure such cases, as I have often observed, not only in my own practice, but in that of others. I have sometimes observed that the first sign of improvement in such cases was a **decided increase in the urine,** and following it a general subsidence of all the other bad symptoms. I have used it with most prompt and satisfactory results in the 1000th (B.& T.) and 33m, (Fincke's) potencies.

Dr. E.B. Nash

HYDRASTIS CAN.: (Constipation) I have found it most efficacious in the 200th (B. & T.). I once cured a case that was of years' standing, had worn cathartics out, and all the way she could live (her words) was to swallow a spoonful of whole flax seed with every meal. I have used it in infantile **constipation successfully,** and it is most useful when **all other symptoms** aside from constipation **are conspicuous for their absence.**

Dr. E.B. Nash

KALIUM BICH.: Of course **leucorrhoeas** of both the ropy and jelly-like variety come under this remedy and many fine cures have resulted from its use.

Dr. E.B. Nash

KALIUM BICH.: I remember one case of years ago in which such **ulcers appeared in the throat of a woman.** One had eaten up through the soft palate into the posterior nares, and the whole palate looked as though it would be destroyed by the **ulcerative process** if not speedily checked. The case had a **syphilitic look** to me and had been under the treatment of two old school physicians for a long time. I gave *Kali bich.* 30th, and to say that I was astonished at the effect (for it was in my early practice) is putting it mildly, for the ulcers healed so rapidly, and her general condition, which was very bad, correspondingly improved, that in three weeks from that time she was well to all appearance and never had any return of the trouble afterwards, or for years, at least as long as I knew her.

Dr. E.B. Nash

KALIUM CARB.: It has cured a number of cases of **fibroid tumors** long before it was the time for the critical period to cure.

You must remember that there is **a natural tendency for a fibroid to cease to grow at the climacteric period,** and afterwards to shrivel and that this takes place without any treatment, but the appropriate remedies will cause that hemorrhage to cease, will cause that tumor to cease to grow and after a few days there will be a shrinkage in its size.

Dr. J.T. Kent

KALIUM CARB.: It is not only a great remedy for **pneumonia, pleurisy** and **heart troubles,** as spoken of, but goes much further and becomes very useful in incipient and even with advanced cases of **phthisis pulmonalis.** I have seen a case pronounced incurable by several old experienced and skillful physicians, Dr. T.L. Brown among them, get well under **a dose once in eight days of Kali carb.**

Dr. E.B. Nash

KALIUM IOD.: '*Kali iod.*' in the words of E.A. Farrington; "**Pneumonia,** in which disease it is an excellent remedy when **hepatization has commenced,** when the disease localizes itself, and infiltration begins. In such cases, in the absence of other symptoms calling distinctively for *Bryonia, Phosphorus* or *Sulphur,* I would advise you to select iodine or *Iodine* of potassa. **It is also called for when** the hepatization is so extensive that we have **cerebral congestion,** or even an **effusion into the brain** as a result of this congestion.

Dr. E.B. Nash

KALIUM MUR.: I have seen enlarged joints after acute rheumatism rapidly reduced to normal size under its action, sometimes after they had resisted other remedies a long time; but I do not know of any characteristic symptoms for its use in preference to other remedies.

Dr. E.B. Nash

KALMIA LAT.: I remember a patient, an old syphilitic, who was told, if he ever made a **violent** move, he would die, **the valves of his heart** were so badly affected. He had all the murmurs that it seemed possible from the heart valves. He had travelled all over and had taken large doses of *Mercury,* and his syphilitic condition had to a great extent been suppressed, until finally the whole trouble had located in the heart. *Kalmia* **removed all the dyspnoea and palpitation in a few months,** and it was nearly two years before, there was a marked return of the symptoms and a repetition put him in a state of health, so that he needed no more medicine. This shows that **what a deep-acting remedy** *Kalmia* **is,** how long it may act, what wonderful change it may effect. A remedy must be capable of going deep into the life to do such things.

Dr. J.T. Kent

LAC CANINUM: Two cases of tonsillitis in one house in separate families, I was called to treat one of them, and a very excellent allopathic physician the other. Of course, there was close watching to see which case would get well the quickest, and especially, if either could be cured without suppuration taking place. They were both very bad cases. Both progressed rapidly for forty-eight hours. **In my case,** the swelling began on one side; the next day was even worse on the other side, so I told them that as the first was better I thought the last one would be better tomorrow; but alas! the **next day number one was worse again,** the patient could not swallow, food and drinks came back by the nose. It was with much difficulty, choking and **struggling that even a spoonful of medicine could be taken.** I hesitated no longer, but gave *Lac caninum* **C.M.** at noon, and when I visited her in the evening, I found her taking oyster broth and she could speak distinctly, whereas she could not articulate a word in the morning. In another day the patient was well except some weakness.

Dr. E.B. Nash

LAC CANINUM: It cured the case very quickly. Not long after I had a very severe case of Scarlatina. The throat was swollen full, and the restlessness was so marked with pains in the limbs which left the patient tossing from side to side that I thought *Rhus tox.* must be the remedy. But it failed to relieve. Then I discovered **that the soreness of the throat and the pains alternated sides.** This called to my mind to the remedy, which was given with **prompt relief. I used the C.M. potency in this case.**

Dr. E.B. Nash

LACHESIS: (ovaritis) H.N. Guernsey: "If pus has already formed **in ovaritis,** *Lachesis* may be the most appropriate remedy to promote its escape externally or through the intestines."

Dr. B. Prasad Gupta

LACHESIS: (action) In many chronic cases its action of **one dose not only lasts for several days,** weeks and months but sometimes one or two doses of *Lachesis* have cured the very chronic and the most complicated cases for ever.

Dr. B. Prasad Gupta

LACHESIS: (Colic) I once had a case of very obstinate constipation in an old syphilitic case. He was at last taken with very severe attacks of colic. The pains seemed to extend all through the abdomen, and always came on at night. After **trying various remedies** until I was discouraged, for he " got no better fast," he let drop this expression, " **Doctor, if I could only keep awake all the time, I would never have another attack.**" I looked askance at him. " I mean," said he, " that I sleep into the attack, and waken in it." I left a dose of *Lachesis* 200. He never had another attack of the pain, and his bowels became perfectly regular from that day and remained so.

Dr. E.B. Nash

LYCOPODIUM: (Cough) It has often saved neglected, mal-treated or imperfectly cured cases of **pneumonia from running into consumption.** It may even come into the later stages of the acute attack itself, and here as usual the disease is apt to be in the **right lung,** and especially if liver complications arise. The disease has passed the first or **congestive stage,** and generally the **stage of hepatization,** or is in the last part of this stage, and is trying hard to take a favourable turn into the breaking up of third stage, the **stage of resolution.** Just here is where many cases die, neither free expectoration, nor **perfect absorption of the disease product taking place. There is extreme dyspnoea,** the cough sounds as if the entire parenchyma of the lung were softened; even raising whole **mouthfuls of mucus does not afford relief,** the breath is short **and the wings of the nose expand to their utmost with a fan-like motion. Now is the time when** *Lycopodium* **does wonders.** Again, even when this stage is imperfectly passed, and the patient still coughs and expectorates much thick, yellow, purulent or grayish-yellow, purulent (sometimes foetid) matter, tasting salty, **with much rattling in the chest,** *Lycopodium* is indispensable.

Dr. E.B. Nash

MERCURIUS SOL.: It cures **lingering febrile conditions** analogous to the typhoid state, but **caused by suppressed ear discharge.** I have cured cases that were due to packing the ear with Borax, Iodoform, etc., the patient having first a remittent and later a continued fever. This would go on for five or six weeks and be relieved only when the discharge returned after a dose of *Mercury.* I remember a case of this type. It was called **cerebrospinal meningitis;** the head was drawn back and twisted and held to one side. It began as on otitis media with **discharge which was suppressed.** Two or three doctors were called and could do nothing. In the night I went to the bedside and got the history and symptoms of *Mercurius. Mercurius* re-established the discharge in twenty-four hours, the torticollis passed away, the fever subsided and the child made an excellent recovery. I can recall many such cases.

Dr. J.T. Kent

MURIATICUM AC.: It cures the muscular weakness following excessive use of opium and tobacco. (*Veratrum alb., Puls., Avena-s., Ipec.*)

Dr. H.C. Allen

MURIATICUM AC.: It is useful in the last **stage of dropsy from Cirrhosis of liver.**

Dr. E.A. Farrington

NATRIUM MUR.: It affects a radical **cure of constipation when many indicated and popular remedies fail.** It is a regulator of water in the system and if moisture is drawn from rectum, loss of function results and produces constipation.

Dr. Heselton

PHOSPHORUS: (Caution) In tuberculosis, it is **oftenest indicated in the incipient stage with the symptom of cough,** oppression and general weakness already mentioned; but I have often found it indicated in the **later stages,** and if given in very high potency and in the **single dose** and not repeated, have seen it greatly benefit even **incurable cases. If given too low and repeated it will fearfully aggravate.**

Dr. E.B. Nash

PLUMBUM MET.: Some years ago a physician came to me in regard to his wife. She had been unconscious for two days and had passed **no urine for days** and the catheter showed that there was **none in the bladder.** She had quite an array of symptoms but they were common symptoms. She had the slowness for days before, and complained of a sensation of continual **pulling at the navel,** as if a string were drawing it back to the spinal column, and then the coma came on. In the middle of the night this doctor came to me in great distress. He said she was pale as death and breathing slow. **A single powder of** *Plumbum* **high potency was given,** and she **passed urine in a few hours,** roused up and never had such an attack again.

Dr. J.T. Kent

PODOPHYLLUM: It is excellent in moderate attacks of **jaundice without fever, in chronic jaundice** not much interfering with the general health.

Dr. Hempel

SILICEA TER.: The child takes nourishment enough, but, whether vomited or retained, **goes on emaciating and growing weaker and weaker until** it dies of inanition, unless *Silicea* checks this process. Many such cases I have saved with this remedy and made them **healthy children**.

Dr. E.B. Nash

SILICEA TER.: It builds them up, and so it seems, for under its action the patient's **spirits rise, hope revives, the weakness and depression given way to a feeling of returning strength** and health. **It makes no difference** whether the ulcerations are in the tissues already named, in the lungs, intestinal track, or mammae, or elsewhere, the effect is the same, and the improvement in the local affection generally follows the general constitutional improvements.

Dr. E.B. Nash

SPIGELIA ANTHE.: I treated in Gumpendorf hospital at Viena, **57 cases of rheumatic carditis** with but one death and *Spigelia* was the **only medicine employed.**

Dr. Flesihman

STICTA PUL.: I have relieved many cases of **chronic catarrh with** *Sticta;* some of years standing.

Dr. E.B. Nash

STRAMONIUM: Once there was a lady about thirty years of age, who was **overheated in the sun,** on an excursion. She was a member in good standing in the Presbyterian church, but imagined herself lost and called for six mornings in succession to see her die. Lost, lost, lost, eternally lost, was her theme, begging minister, doctor and everybody to pray for, and with her. **Talked night and day** about it. I had to shut her up in her room alone for she would not sleep a wink or let anyone else.

She imagined her head was as big as a bushel and had me examine her legs, which she insisted were as large as a church. **After treating her several weeks with** *Glonoine,* *Lach., Natrum carb.* and other remedies on the cause as the basis of the prescription, without the least amelioration of her condition, **I gave her** *Stramonium,* **which covered her symptoms,** and in twenty-four hours every vertigo of that mania was gone. But for the encouragement, I told the husband that I could cure her. She would have been sent to the Utica asylum, where her friends had been advised to send her by the allopaths. **I gave her the sixth dilution** or potency.

Dr. E.B. Nash

STRAMONIUM: The whole inner mouth as if raw; the **tongue after a while may become stiff or paralyzed.** Stools loose, blackish, smelling like carrion, or **no stool or urine.** Later there may be complete **loss of sight, hearing,** and speech with dilated, immovable pupils and **drenching sweat** which brings no relief, and death must soon close the scene unless Stramonium helps them out.

Dr. E.B. Nash

SULPHUR: Your former remedy was well chosen and seemed to help the patient in a measure, but the **case relapses, lingers or progresses slowly to perfect recovery. It is on account of a depression of the vital force,** as Hahnemann would call it. It may be on account of psora or not. Now give a dose of *Sulphur* and **let it act a few hours if in an acute case, or a number of days if chronic.** Then you may return to your former remedy and get results which you could not get before the *Sulphur* was given. **It clears up the case and prevents its becoming chronic or a lingering,**

unsatisfactory convalescence.

Dr. E.B. Nash

SULPHUR: (Skin and Stomach) A lady (maiden) had been an invalid for fourteen years. Her trouble seemed to **centre in her stomach.** So that for all that long period of time she could eat nothing but a little graham bread and milk, hardly enough to sustain life, and in the earlier part of her sickness for a long time was able **only to take a teaspoonful of milk at a time.** She was an almost literal **walking skeleton.** I found, after much questioning and several failures to relieve her much, that about fifteen years before she had, with an **ointment suppressed an eczema** of the nape and occiput. She boasted that she had never seen a vertigo of it since. **I gave that lady Sulphur 200 and in three weeks from that time** had that **eruption** fully restored and her stomach trouble completely relieved.

Dr. E.B. Nash

TUBERCULINUM BOV.: Dr. Swan cured a case of **headache of forty-five years standing with Tuberculinum.**

Dr. B. Prasad Gupta

TUBERCULINUM: In view of what Dr. Burnett has written, and my own limited experience lately, I am confident that *Tuberculinum* is destined to rank with *Psorinum* in the treatment of **chronic disease.**

Dr. E.B. Nash

USTILAGO MAY.: *Ustilago maydis* has cured negro *Urticaria* of six years standing.

Dr. B. Prasad Gupta

VERATRUM ALB.: If we were to describe in one word the general condition, as near as possible, for which this remedy was best, it would be **collapse.** Let me quote: " **Rapid sinking of forces; complete prostration; cold sweat and cold breath."** "Skin blue, purple, cold, wrinkled, remaining in folds when pinched." "Face Hippocratic; nose pointed." "Whole body icy cold." "Cold skin, face cold, back cold." "Hands icy cold." "Feet and legs icy cold." (icy coldness of surface, covered with cold sweat, *Tabacum.*) **"Cramps in Calves."** All these are verified symptoms, and show to what an extreme degree of collapse a case may come and yet be cured. This condition may be found in rapidly progressing, acute cases like cholera, or it may be found in suppressed exanthemata; or , again, in the course of bronchitis, pneumonia, typhoid or intermittent fever. **No matter where found, or in connection with whatever disease, if this collapse is present, and especially if the grand keynote, " cold sweat on face and forehead," is present,** we may give this remedy with full confidence that it will do all that can be done and much more than the old school system of stimulation with alcoholics.

Dr. E.B. Nash

ZINCUM MET.: A young lady about 20 years of age complained, a week before I was called, of weakness, or feeling of general prostration; headache, and loss of appetite, but the greatest complaint was of **prostration.** She was a student and her mother, who was an excellent nurse, attributed all her sickness to overwork at school, and tried to rest and " nurse her up." but she continued to grow worse. **I prescribed** for her *Gelsemium* and followed it with *Bryonia* **according to indications,** and she ran through a mild course of two weeks longer, and seemed convalescing quite satisfactorily.

Being left in a room alone, while sleeping and perspiring, she threw off her clothes, caught cold and relapsed. Of course the "last stage of that patient was worse than the first." The bowels became enormously distended, profuse hemorrhage occurred, which was **finally controlled by** *Alumen,* a low form of delirium came on, the prostration became extreme notwithstanding the hemorrhage was checked, until the following picture obtained, **staring eyes** rolled upward into the head, head retracted; complete unconsciousness, lying on back and sliding down in bed, twitching, or rather intense, violent trembling all over, so that she shook the bed. I had **nurses to hold her hands night and day, she shook** and trembled so; Hippocratic face, extremities deathly cold to knees and elbows, pulse so weak and quick I could not count it, and intermittent; in short, all signs of **impending paralysis of the brain. The case seemed hopeless, but I put ten drops of** *Zincum metallicum* **in two drams of cold water,** and worked one-half of its between her set teeth, a little at a time, and an hour after the other half. About one hour after the last dose she turned her eyes down and faintly said, "milk." Through a bent tube she swallowed a half glass of milk, the first nourishment she had received in 24 hours. She got no more medicine for four days, and improved steadily all the time. She, afterward received **a dose of** *Nux vomica* and progressed rapidly to a perfect recovery. So *Zincum* 200 **can, like other metals, perform miracles when indicated.**

Dr. E.B. Nash

6. HOMEOPATHY
vs.
ALLOPATHY

CROTON TIG.: When the allopaths, in any case where they considered an operation of the bowels imperative, had exhausted all other resources, *Croton tiglium* was their "biggest gun for the last broadside." In other words, this is a most **violent cathartic.** Now if similia, etc., is not true, Croton tig. ought utterly **to fail to cure diarrhea;** but it is true, and not withstanding this remedy has proved its truth over and over again the allopaths deny and reject homeopathy.

Dr. E.B. Nash

IPECACUANHA: (Loose prescribing) I have cured many cases of fever and ague by the first prescription, thus saving myself a good deal of unnecessary seeking and comparing. Whatever may be said in **condemnation of this loose prescribing, it is certainly preferable to the inevitable** *Quinine* prescription of the old school, and some self-styled homeopaths, for the reason that it will cure more cases than *Quinine,* and do infinitely less harm. *Ipecac.* can cure more cases than quinine, but both can cure the case to which they are homeopathic, and that in the potentized form of the drug. **We have such clear-cut indications for the use of many remedies that we need not fail once where the allopaths do twenty times, with their** indiscriminate Quinine treatment.

Dr. Jahr

OPIUM: This is the reason why the homeopath can make his sleepless patient sleep **a natural sleep with** *Opium* **in the little dose,** while the allopath forces his patient into a stupor (not a sleep) with his big dose. The one is curative, the other poisonous.

Dr. E.B. Nash

PLATINUM MET.: I was led by it to prescribe the remedy in a very **obstinate case of insanity** which had resisted the skill of several allopathic physicians of note, and they had finally decided that the case must be sent to the insane asylum. The parents, however, who were quite wealthy, could not consent to that, and were induced to try homeopathy. I gave her *Platina* on the strength of this mental indication, which was very prominent, coupled with another prominent symptom, which also appears under this remedy, viz., **"physical symptoms disappear when mental symptoms appear,"** and vice versa. This physical symptom was **a pain in the whole length of the spine.** This was the symptom alternating with the mental one. It was one of the most brilliant cures I ever saw. Improvement began the first day and never flagged, and she remained well now 15 years, with never a sign of return.

Dr. E.B. Nash

■

7. PATHOLOGY
AND
SYMPTOMATOLOGY

CANCER

What is the Scirrhus but a peculiar form of induration! When the economy takes on a low type of life, a low form of tissue making, and the tissues inflame and upon the slightest provocation, **indurate,** we can see that this is a kind of constitution that is predisposed to deep-seated troubles, to phthisis, Bright's disease, diabetes, cancer etc.

Dr. J.T. Kent

CEREBELLUM

The cerebellum presides over respiration during **sleep** and the cerebrum presides over respiration when the patient is **awake.**

Dr. J.T. Kent

HEART-HOPELESSNESS; LUNG-HOPELESSNESS

With every little trouble located in the **heart,** there comes **hopelessness,** but when the manifestation of disease is in the **lungs,** there is **hopefulness.**

Dr. J.T. Kent

HYDROCEPHALOID CASE

The first permanent and substantial indication that the remedy is working in a **Hydrocephaloid** case is that it increases the **flow of urine,** which has been scanty all the time.

Dr. J.T. Kent

HYPERTENSION

It must be remembered that chronic **renal infection** is an important cause of hypertension.

Dr. Kesav Pai

INSOMNIA

I consider *Gelsemium* 1x one of our best remedies for insomnia and there are no bad after effects.

Dr. Kuthbert

LATE MARRIAGE AND LABOUR

Woman who marries at 28 or 30, or later, suffer from **prolonged labor.**

Dr. J.T. Kent

PATHOLOGY

It seems to me like folly, to undertake, to pose as either an exclusive pathologist or symptomatologist. **Both pathology and symptomatology** are valuable and inseparable; neither can be excluded. Pathology is what the **doctor can tell** (sometimes); symptomatology is what the **patient can tell.**

Dr. E.B. Nash

PRESCRIBING IN HOMEOPATHY

I only tell you this to give you an idea how long it takes to restore order, for nature herself to replace the bad tissue and put healthy tissue in that same place, to restore an organ. It takes time, and it is best that we should not be surprised. It may be that the medicine has done all it can do. Here is another thing I have seen; even when there were no symptoms left, and after waiting a considerable time, there were no symptoms. I have seen that another dose of the same medicine that was given on the last symptoms, give the patient a great lift, and pathological conditions commence to go away. So *Calcarea* is a great friend to the oculist, and every physician ought to be just as good a prescriber as the oculist can be, for he prescribes for the patient. So must the oculist. In prescribing, I am in doubt whether there can be any such thing as a speciality, because the homeopathic physician prescribes for the patient. **He prescribes for the patient, whether he has eye disease, ear disease, throat disease, lung disease, or liver disease, etc.**

Dr. J.T. Kent

Rains Aggravate

One of the most characteristic symptoms of the *Elaps* proving is the marked aggravation from rain or the approach of rain, the aggravation from rain or its approach in *Elaps* **out generals this symptoms in Rhus tox.**

Dr. H.A. Roberts

Sprain

Immediately **bathing with water as hot as can be borne** for length of time, followed by a compress of *Arnica, Aconite,*

Rhus tox. or *Ruta.* This treatment, employed promptly, generally **cures at once.**

Dr. Ruddock

Thirst

Phosphorus, although it has the marked symptom of **unquenchable thirst** for cold drinks, also, is a **thirstless** remedy, a fact which is very easily overlooked.

Dr. Rudolph F. Rabe

TOWARDS CURE

Do not be discouraged in prescribing **if the pathological** conditions do not go away; but if all the symptoms of the patient have gone away, and the patient is eating well, and is sleeping well, and doing well, do not feel that it is impossible for that opacity of the cornea to go away, for sometimes it will.

Dr. J.T. Kent

APIS MEL.: There is scarcely a remedy that has such marked symptoms of **glossitis** as *Apis.*

British Journal of Homeopathy

BELLADONNA: Guernsey says: "This medicine is particularly applicable, and in fact takes the lead over all others in cases in which quickness or suddenness of either sensation or motion is predominant." To be sure all these symptoms have their pathological explanation if we could give it; but, acting on our law of similia, we can cure our patients and are not left at sea, without chart or compass, because we cannot explain. We know that these symptoms

are the **natural outcome of the pathological state,** and that
the administration of a poison which is capable of setting up
a similar outcome, cures the patient.

Dr. E.B. Nash

NUX VOM.: As regards **to side affected** in *Nux vomica,*
abdominal symptoms find to be right sided, and chest
symptoms left sided.

Dr. D.M. Gibson

OPIUM: I know some people who are made absolutely
sleepless by opium in all sorts of doses, and *Opium* 30 has
helped me in **cases of sleeplessness,** as often as *Coffea.*

Dr. J.H. Clarke

PODOPHYLLUM PELT.: All drugs have their double
action, or what is called **primary and secondary** action. But
the surest and most lasting curative action of any drug is
that in which the condition to be cured **simulates the primary**
action of the drug. For, as I have held elsewhere, I think that
what is called **secondary** action of the drug is really not the
legitimate action of drug but the **aroused powers of the
organism against the drug.** So, the alternate diarrhea and
constipation in disease is a fight, for instance, between the
disease (diarrhea) and the **natural powers resisting it.** It is
of considerable importance then to be able to recognize in
such a case whether it is the diarrhea or constipation that is
the disease, against which the alternate condition is the effort
of the **vital force** to establish health. Yet such an
understanding is not always absolutely imperative, for in
either case there are generally enough concomitant

symptoms to decide the choice of the remedy. Indeed, the choice must always rest upon either the peculiar and characteristic symptoms appearing in the case or the totality of them. None, but the true homeopathist learns to appreciate this. Here is, where, what is called pathological prescribing often fails, for the choice of the **remedy may depend upon symptoms entirely outside of the symptoms** which go to make up the pathology of the case, at least so far as we understand pathology.

Dr. E.B. Nash

SEPIA: It is essential to ascertain the **seat of the local disease** with accuracy; for, every experienced homeopath knows how in **toothache for instance,** it is necessary to select the remedy, which in its proving has repeatedly acted upon the **very tooth that suffers.**

The specific curative power of *Sepia* in those stubborn and sometimes **fatal joint abscesses** evidence upon this point, for they differ from similar gatherings in location only, **while the remedies so suitable for abscess elsewhere remain ineffectual here.**

Dr. C.M. Boger

∎

8. AGGRAVATIONS — WHICH ARE MEANINGFUL

ARSENICUM ALB.: In psoriasis, the first influence of *Arsenicum* is to make the **eruption redder and more inflamed**. This fact **if not known,** would lead to the suspension of the medicine just when it commenced to do good; at the same time, it is unnecessary to give it in doses sufficiently large to do this.

Dr. Ringer

CONIUM MAC.: I once treated a case of what seemed to be **locomotor ataxia** with this remedy.

The patient had been slowly **losing the use of his legs; could not stand in the dark;** and when he walked along the street, would make his wife walk either ahead of him, or behind him, for the act of looking sidewise, for in the least turning, head or eyes that way would cause him to stagger or fall. **Conium cured him. It would always aggravate at first, but he would greatly improve after stopping the remedy.** The aggravation was just as invariable after taking a dose of Fincke's cm. potency as from anything lower, but the improvement lasted longer after it. Taking an **occasional dose** from a week to four weeks apart completely cured him in about a year. It was a bad case, of years standing, before I took him.

Dr. E.B. Nash

HYOSCYAMUS NIG.: It is very useful in a **form of dry cough which** is aggravated **when lying** down and relieved by sitting up.

Dr. E.B. Nash

KALIUM CARB.: All the Kalis are aggravated after any disturbance in fluid balance in the body, **particularly after coition.**

Dr. Donald A. Davis

LYCOPODIUM: It will throw out a greater amount of eruption at first, but this will subside finally and the child will return to health.

Dr. J.T. Kent

MEDORRHINUM: (Rheumatism) I have experimented more with the so-called **nosodes** and I have seemingly very good results from this remedy as well as *Syphilinum* in intractable cases of **chronic rheumatism.** The most characteristic difference between them is that with *Medorrhinum* the pains are worse in the **day-time,** and with *Syphilinum* **in the night.**

Dr. E.B. Nash

NATRIUM MUR.: In dropsy after the malaria *Natrum mur.*, when it acts curatively, generally **brings back the original chill.**

Dr. J.T. Kent

SEPIA: This is to be **given in the evening because** if given in the morning, it may produce a sufficient aggravation to leave the patient feeling quite, unless for that day.

Dr. R.A.F. Jack

SULPHUR: When a patient is aggravated by *Sulphur*, we must always think of the existence of a latest state of Syphilis, if *Pulsatilla,* another antidote of *Sulphur* does not produce any result.

Dr. Leon Renard

SULPHUR: So strong is this **affinity** of *Sulphur* for the skin that it seems bent on **pushing** everything internal, **out on the surface.**

Dr. E.B. Nash

VERATURM ALB.: It is said to be a good remedy for **rheumatism,** which is worse in **wet weather** and which drives the patient out of bed.

Dr. E.B. Nash

ZINCUM MET.: A tedious aggravation in the **convulsion** and fever and a continuous **brain cry** is to be expected if a perfect cure is to result with the administration of *Zincum met.*

Dr. J.T. Kent

AFTER RELIEF

After a prescription, giving relief, **do not give** a remedy **for any new symptoms** appearing in a less vital part.

Dr. Adolph Lippe

THREE DOSES

You can **avoid aggravation** from high potency by giving it three doses two hours apart.

Dr. T.K. Moore

OBSERVATIONS

It is prime rule **not to keep repeating** your remedy **when** the intervals between aggravations of the disease are lengthening. This is an indication that the patient is improving.

Homeo Recorder, Aug.31

THE TWO CONTEMPORARY STARS!
(IN HOMEOPATHY)

Homeopathy has seen two shining starts in the same period - with marked difference in their personalities.

1. Nash was devoted mostly to practice and individualized patients, Kent generalized many things and established principles for the generation.

2. Nash was a bit emotional in his expressions; Kent was more a philosopher.

3. Nash was not very conscious about people around; Kent was extremely conscious of the society and how people felt.

(Both lost their sight in the last phase of their life.)

(Quoted from "Two Stars of Homeopathy" by the Author)

9. CAUTIONS IN HOMEOPATHY

ACHIEVEMENTS-INCOMPLETE

There may be conditions in the human race that we, as yet, know no remedy for. We see certain groups of peculiar symptoms frequently repeat themselves and we know they are representatives of a state of the economy, but up to this day, we may not have seen in the **Materia Medica, their counterpart. In medicines, we have the exact counterpart for the diseases of the human race.**

Dr. J.T. Kent

ACUTE CASES

In acute cases, one must have a remedy of the highest rating in the outstanding symptoms.

Dr. J. Stephenson

ACUTE REMEDY

All the symptoms should be examined between the attacks, so that the child may be elevated above these attacks, because the acute remedy **will do no more than suit the first, or second, or third at the most.**

Dr. J.T. Kent

ANAEMIA

The general practitioner confronted with a case exhibiting anaemia must **avoid the temptation to commence treatment** before making a diagnosis, for even single dose of haematinic may entirely alter the marrow picture within twenty four hours.

Dr. Charles Seward

ANTI-PSORIC

The best time for taking an anti-psoric is in the **morning** before breakfast.

Dr. Samuel Hahnemann

Anti-psorics are apt to do harm in **active Syphilis,** i.e. as long as the Syphilis is the upper most miasm. But many anti-psorics are also anti-syphilitics, and they are not to be excluded as a rule.

Dr. J.T. Kent

ASPIRIN

I stress the great danger of Aspirin and all Aspirin type drugs, even Alka-Seltzer, in people liable to **peptic ulcer.** Every year, we see at least one case and sometimes two or three with quite severe haematemesis from this cause, often requiring transfusion. The risk is especially great in febrile states, influenza etc., where gastritis is already present, and Aspirin sets up acute ulcerations not demonstrable on x-rays but capable of **causing even fatal haemorrhage.**

Dr. T.D. Ross

CAUTION

In **enteric fever,** when the temperature comes down to normal and even sub-normal, without any serious condition, don't give a remedy, **since** that will cause relapse.

Dr. Boger

DANGER AHEAD

Whenever treating a severe form of disease and an **eruption** comes to the surface, like a carbuncle or erysipelas, and does **not give relief to the patient ,then there is danger.** A remedy must be found soon.

Dr. J.T. Kent

DANGEROUS REMEDIES

Phosphorus, Silicea and *Lachesis* are three very dangerous remedies, if there is **pre-tubercular tendency.** The wrong potency or too frequent repetition may drive the patient into an active Tuberculosis.

Dr. E.W. Hubbard

GALL STONES

I am never very happy about **leaving gall stones,** specially **if the gall bladder is inflamed** because of the danger of gall stone ileus. A stone ulcerating through into the duodenum, may pass down the small intestine causing great damage and a most cheating type of intestinal intermittent obstruction often leading to gangrene of a large section of the bowel.

Dr. T.D. Rose

INCUBATION PERIOD

It is well-known fact that **any sort of prophylactic,** potentised or crude, falling within the **incubation period** of any infection, often, not only fails, but leads to virulent and even fatal aggravation.

Dr. J.N. Kanjilal

INIMICALS

Most of the symptoms in *Causticum* are aggravated from **drinking coffee.** You should therefore not allow patients to drink this beverage while taking *Causticum.*

Dr. Boger

'Coffee' **must never be used when** *Chamomilla* or *Nux* is the remedy. It would be equally true if you are treating a nervous paralytic with *Causticum.*

Dr. J.T. Kent

NOSODE

When a **nosode comes** out in repertorizing, use it with care. It proves to be the similimum.

Dr. James Stephenson

PREGNANCY

Apis should be **cautiously** given during first three **months of pregnancy** in low potencies, as it is liable to produce miscarriages.

Dr. Cowperthwaite

PRESCRIBING CORRECTLY

After a prescription giving relief, do not give a remedy for any new symptoms appearing in a less vital part.

Dr. Adolph Lippe

REPETITION

Always conserve the strength of your patient and never repeat a remedy which **exhausts him.**

Homeo. Recorder, Aug.31

REPETITION-WITH CARE !

The routine prescriber gives *Belladonna* to a child who has hot head, hot face and throbbing carotids and when it does not help he gives more Belladonna, and increases the **size of his dose until the child has a proving.**

Dr. J.T. Kent

RESTLESS REMEDIES

Rhus tox. and *Arsenicum alb.* are often indicated in typhoids, *Aconite* seldom or never, but all three are equally **restless remedies.**

Dr. E.B. Nash

SELECTION

Sometimes a very poor prescriber may hunt around and get one remedy for one group of symptoms and other remedy for another group, and the patient becomes worse than before. If the remedies are similar as to **their general nature, then,** the little superficial symptoms are not so extremely important.

Dr. J.T. Kent

WAIT-WHEN IMPROVEMENT

The safe rule is, where there is definite and continuous improvement, nature has got the matter in hand, so just put yours behind you till the reappearance of symptoms demand further attention.

Dr. M.L. Tyler

ACONITUM NAP.: The custom of alternating *Aconite* and *Belladonna* in inflammatory affections, which so widely prevails, is a senseless one. Both remedies cannot be indicated at a time, and if a good effect follows their administration, you may be sure that the indicated one cured in spite of the action of the other, which only hindered; or that the patient recovered without help from either

Dr. E.B. Nash

ACONITUM NAP.: So-called homeopaths have fallen into similar ERROR by concluding that, because *Aconite* did quickly cure in some cases having a high grade of fever, that therefore it was always the remedy with which to treat cases having fever. They even fall into the routine habit of prescribing this remedy for the first stage of all inflammatory affections, and follow it with other remedies more appropriate to the whole case further on.

Dr. E.B. Nash

ACONITUM NAP.: *Aconite* is never to be given first to subdue the fever and then some other remedy 'to meet the case,' never to be alternated with other drugs for the purpose, as is often alleged of 'controlling the fever.' If the fever be such as to require *Aconite*, no other drug is needed. If other drugs seem indicated, one should be soughted out, which meets the fever as well, for many drugs besides *Aconite* produce fever, each of its kind."

Dr. Carrol Dunham

QUININE SUPPRESSES

ARSENICUM ALB.: *Arsenicum* is one of our best remedies for fevers of a typhoid character. So useful is it that **Baehr says:** "since *Arsenic* is, more than any other remedy, adapted to the worst forms of infectious diseases, it seems wrong to delay its administration until the symptoms indicating it are developed in their most malignant intensity," and further, 'our advice, therefore, is that *Arsenic* should be given more frequently than has been customary from the very beginning of the attack, and that we should not wait until the disease has fully developed its pernicious character." **I do not think, this is sound reasoning** or good advice, for I have never found any rule by which I could decide from the beginning that a case would later on develop into a case of a pernicious or malignant character which would ever call for the exhibition of *Arsenic*. While we need not wait for a case to develop to that "most malignant" intensity which calls for *Arsenic* **we would not, on the other hand be justified in giving** *Arsenic* **or any other remedy in anticipation of a condition which might never come.** *Arsenicum* is not the only remedy capable of curing these malignant cases, and how do we know after all that it may not be *Muriatic acid* or *Carbo veg.* that will be the remedy after the case is developed. **There is no safe or scientific rule but to treat the case with the indicated remedy** at any and all stages of the disease, without trying to treat expected conditions or future possibilities.

Dr. E.B. Nash

BERBERIS VUL.: The remedy that is indicated for the patient will **cure the patient, and the fistula.** Above all things, they should not be operated on. **To close up that fistulous opening, and thus neglect the patient, is a very dangerous thing to do.** Knowing all that I know, if such a trouble would come upon me and I could not find the remedy to cure it, I would near with it patiently, knowing I was keeping a much less grievance. Nor could I advise my patient to have a thing done that I would not have done upon myself. It is a dangerous thing to operate upon fistula. It is a very serious matter. **If it is closed up, and that patient is leaning towards phthisis,** he will develop phthisis; if he has a tendency towards Bright's disease, that will hasten it; if he threatens to break down in any direction, his weakest parts will be affected, and he will break down. Occasionally enough time elapses so that the physician who is ignorant does not see the relation between the two. But now that you have heard it, you can never forget it.

Dr. J.T. Kent

BRYONIA ALB.: When patients are under constitutional remedies, they need **caution about certain kinds of food that are** known to disagree with their constitutional remedy. A Bryonia patient is often **made sick from eating sauer kraut, from vegetable salads, chicken salad, etc.,** so that you need not be surprised, after administering a dose of *Bryonia* for a constitutional state, to have your patient come in and say she has been made very ill from eating some one of these things. **It is well to caution persons** who are under the influence of *Pulsatilla* to avoid the use of fatty foods, because very often they will upset the action of the remedy which is similar to the patient when you administer it, and the things that he is to have are to be in agreement with that remedy.

Dr. J.T. Kent

CHINA: The sugar pills cure safely, permanently and gently, while the quinine never cures, but **suppresses,** and there is nothing in the history of that patient drugged with quinine and arsenic but congestion and violence so long as he lives.

Dr. J.T. Kent

COCCUS CACTI: If patient can lie in a **cool room without much covering** he will go **longer without coughing.**

Dr. J.T. Kent

EUPATORIUM PERF.: The time for the administration of this dose is at the **close of the paroxysm.** You get the best effect when reaction is at the best, that is when reaction is setting in, after a paroxysm has passed off. That is true of every paroxysmal disease, when it is possible to wait until the end.

Dr. J.T. Kent

BE WARE !

It is better to know what you have done if you have killed your patient, than to be ignorant of it and go on and kill some more in the same way.

Dr. J.T. Kent

FERRUM MET.: If you are treating a case of Syphilis with gumma in the brain where it is likely to be present in the later stage of syphilis, *Ferrum* might produce apoplexy, because of the already friable condition of the blood vessels. **Then avoid *Ferrum* in** Tuberculosis, Syphilis and in persons predisposed to haemorrhages and especially never repeat it.

Dr. J.T. Kent

FERRUM MET.: Iron is no more a panacea for anaemia than is quinine for malaria or phosphate of lime for deficient bone development. My experience has taught me that there are several other equally efficient remedies for these conditions and that when they are not indicated they not only cannot cure **but do harm every time they** are prescribed, especially in the material doses in which they are generally recommended by such teachers. I must here state my experience founded on abundant practice and observation that, such prescribing is not only un-Hahnemannian, but in every sense **unhomeopathic,** and I warn all beginners not to practice along that line or they too **will come to talk of** the few satisfactory and certain things in modern medicine.

Dr. E.B. Nash

HELLEBORUS NIG.: When it was given, repair set in; not instantly, but **gradually,** the remedy acts slowly in slow, stubborn, stupid cases of **brain and spinal trouble.** Sometimes, there is no apparent change until the day after the remedy is administered or even the next night, when there comes a **sweat, a diarrhea, or vomiting**—a reaction. **They must not be interfered with, no remedy must be given.** They are signs of reaction. If the child has vitality enough to recover, he will now recover. **If the vomiting is stopped by any remedy that will stop it, the Helleborus will be antidoted.**

Dr. J.T. Kent

HEPAR SULPH: If our medicines were not powerful enough to **kill folks,** they would not be powerful enough to **cure sick folks.** It is well, for you to realize that you are dealing with razors, when **dealing with high potencies.** I would rather be in a room **with a dozen negroes slashing with razors than in the hands of an ignorant prescriber of high potencies.** They are means of **tremendous harm**, as well as of tremendous good.

Dr. J.T. Kent

HEPAR SULPH: It is only very rarely that you will be able with your medicines, to cure a stricture after it has taken on permanency, after it is many years old, **but as long as the inflammation keeps up there is hope.**

Dr. J.T. Kent

HYOSCYAMUS NIGER: It is also very **useful in scarlatina of the typhoid form,** and is **complementary to Rhus tox.** in those cases. **I never alternate the two,** but if the depressed sensorium and delirium goes beyond the power of *Rhus tox.* to control, I suspend the *Rhus tox.* for a day or two and give *Hyoscyamus,* which will so improve the case that *Rhus tox.* may again come into use and carry it to a successful termination. **This is the only alternation I am ever guilty of. It is like that of Hahnemann, when he alternated** *Bryonia* and *Rhus* in fevers.

Dr. E.B. Nash

IGNATIA: It is best to administer the dose in the **morning if there is no occasion for hurry;** when given shortly before bed time, it causes too much restlessness at night.

Dr. Samuel Hahnemann

IODIUM: The local application for **glandular enlargement** is foolish and dangerous.

Dr. E.B. Nash

KALIUM CARB.: In old gouty cases, in old cases of Bright's disease, in advanced cases of phthisis where there are many tubercles, **beware of Kali carb. given too high.**

Dr. J.T. Kent

LAC DEF.: Many people **are made sick by milk** who use cream with safety and delight. Lac defloratum is often the remedy for such patients and after a careful examination, their symptoms appear like the proving of skimmed milk.

Dr. J.T. Kent

LACHESIS: It is recommended in **epilepsy** and locomotor ataxia, **but I have never seen good effects from it.**

Dr. E.B. Nash

NUX VOMICA: *Nux vomica* will neither antidote the effects of the drug poison nor cure the disease condition, **unless it is homeopathically indicated, especially if given in the dynamic form.**

Dr. E.B. Nash

NUX VOMICA: No physician would be justified in prescribing *Nux vomica* on temperament alone, be the indication ever so clear. **The whole case must come in.**

Dr. E.B. Nash

NUX VOMICA: *Nux vomica* acts best when **given at night,** during repose of mind and body; *Sulphur* in the morning.

Dr. E.B. Nash

OPIUM: There is **no response to light, touch, noise or anything else,** except the indicated remedy, which is *Opium.* So, in pneumonia, where *Opium* has made remarkable cures in homeopathic hand; while in massive, or what they like to call heroic, doses of the old school (given to stop pain and procure sleep), it has **sent many a poor victim to his long resting place.**

Dr. E.B. Nash

PHOSPHORUS: The deeper remedies ought to be avoided if the vital force is low. Hahnemann warned against the use of *Phosphorus* in such cases of **deficient vitality.**

Dr. J.T. Kent

PHOSPHORUS: Beware of giving it in impotency or in weakness, as this is often associated with very feeble constitutions, and *Phosphorus* not only fails to cure, but seems **to add to the weakness.** *Phosphorus* will set patients to running down more rapidly, who are suffering from vital weakness, who are always tired, simply weak, always prostrated and want to go to bed.

Dr. J.T. Kent

PSORINUM: Psorinum patient does not improve while **coffee is taken.**

Dr. P. Banerjee

RHUS TOX: *Rhus tox.* is no less valuable in **chronic skin** troubles than in **acute. Eczemas** of the vesicular type are often cured by it; there is much itching which is not greatly relieved by scratching.

Dr. E.B. Nash

KALI CARB: It would sometimes be cruel to give a dose of *Kali carb.* **when the colic is on,** because if the remedy fitted the case constitutionally, if all the symptoms of the case were those of *Kali carb.,* you would be **likely to get an aggravation,** that would be unnecessary. There are plenty of short acting remedies that would relieve the pain speedily, and at the close of the attack the constitutional remedy could then be given.

Dr. J.T. Kent

KALIUM CARB.: Do not be afraid to give the anti-psoric remedies when there is a history of tuberculosis in the family, but be careful when the patient is so far advanced with tuberculosis that there are cavities in the lung, or latent tubercles, or encysted caseous tubercles, and some day after, practicing while and making numerous mistakes in **attempting to cure incurables,** you will admit the awful power of homeopathic medicines.

Dr. J.T. Kent

PODOPHYLLUM: It is a common feature after giving a high potency of *podophyllum* in a diarrhea, that a headache comes on after the diarrhea is stopped, it means that the medicine has acted suddenly and the **headache will pass away soon.**

Dr. J.T. Kent

RUMEX CRIS.: If the diarrhea is very exhausting, use some simple medicine, like this one, to slack it up. **But the phthisical patient is better off with a little diarrhea,** a loose morning stool. It is the same with night sweat; if he does not have them he will have something more violent.

Dr. J.T. Kent

RUMEX CRIS.: In advanced cases of phthisis with early morning diarrhea, when *Sulphur* is indicated but which aggravates if given, this medicine is useful.

Dr. J.T. Kent

SECALE COR.: I fully agree with Cowperthwaite, who says: "to give it in parturition to hasten delivery, as is the practice of the old school, is simply inexcusable." On the other hand, I agree with **Dr. H.N. Guernsey,** "that it is useful when labor pains are weak, suppressed or distressing, in weak, cachectic women, in the 200th dilution," and have verified it beyond question.

Dr. E.B. Nash

SECALE COR.: **Weak pains** remedied by the indicated homeopathic drug bring on **natural labor,** while large doses for the same purpose of an unindicated one do not and never can produce natural labor. It is nothing more or less than **drug poisoning.**

Dr. E.B. Nash

SILICEA: There are cases that would be greatly injured by so deep acting remedy as *Silicea,* if given **in the beginning,** i.e, the suffering would be unnecessary; but **if you commence with *Pulsatilla,* you can mitigate the case and prepare it to receive *Silicea,*** providing the two would appear to be on a plane of agreement. A very serious case had better first receive *Pulsatilla,* and the way being paved by that remedy, follow it up with *Silicea.*

Dr. J.T. Kent

■

10. COMPLEMENTARY AND INIMICALS

ALTERNATION

COFFEA CRUDA: Hering used to recommend *Aconite* and *Coffea* in alternation in painful inflammatory affections, where the fever symptoms of the former and also the nervous sensibility of the latter were present, and **I know of no two remedies that alternate better, though I never do it, since I learned to closely individualize.**

Dr. E.B. Nash

ANTIDOTES

Cadmium sulph and *Phosphorus* **are antidotes** to *Radium brom.*, in case of treatment of *Carcinoma* by radiation. Give 1M.

Dr. R.B. Das

COLIC

Colocynthis cures colics again and again. Then *Kali carb.* steps to **end the troubles.**

Dr. T.K. Moore

COMPLEMENTARY

Silicea is the **chronic** of *Pulsatilla.*

Dr. E.B. Nash

China and *Carbo veg.* are **decidedly** complementary

Dr. E.B. Nash

RELATIONSHIP

I should give *Causticum* after *Phosphorus, Silicea* after *Mercury,* or *Rhus tox.* after *Apis mel.*, **if I found them indicated.**

Dr. E.B. Nash

REPETITION

When the remedy is not similar enough to cure in such a form, the **increasing of the dose does not make it homeopathic.** There is an idea in vogue that increasing the dose makes the remedy similar. That is going away from principle. If the remedy is not similar there is no form of dose that can make it similar.

Dr. J.T. Kent

SEQUENCE

If *Coffea* does not relieve, **follow with** *Chamomilla.*

Dr. E.B. Nash

PSORINUM is often **indicated** after Pyrogen.

Dr. E. Underhill

ARGENTUM NIT.: *Cuprum metallicum* has great restlessness between the attacks. Finally, *Natrum muriaticum* is the best **antidote** for the abuse of *Argentums nit.*, especially upon mucus surfaces.

Dr. E.B. Nash

ARSENICUM ALB.: It often **follows well** after *Mercurius*, if that remedy only partially relieves.

Dr. E.B. Nash

CALCAREA OST.: It is one of the most effective agents, if indicated by the **temperament and symptoms,** in the cure of pulmonary consumption, and if applied at a stage when the cure is at all possible.

Dr. E.B. Nash

CARBO VEG.: Acidity and pyrosis is frequent; the **plainest food disagrees,** fatty foods especially. Here *Carbo veg.* succeeds when *Pulsatilla* fails.

Dr. E.B. Nash

CARBO VEG.: *China* is its great complementary.

Dr. E.B. Nash

COLCHICUM AUT.: It is always set down in the text-books for **rheumatism**, articular, migrating and gouty diseases and I have often tried it, but **never with anything like the success** of our other rheumatic remedies. I have been greatly disappointed in it here.

Dr. E.B. Nash

FERRUM MET.: (anaemia) It is evident, therefore, that **iron does not act as a curative agent by virtue of its absorption** as a constituent of the blood, but rather, as we are led to conclude, from its physiological effects upon the organs and tissues of the body, that it owes its therapeutic virtues to the same essential dynamic agency possessed by other drugs, and its application is subject to the same therapeutic law.

Dr. E.B. Nash

IGNATIA AMAR.: *Ignatia* bears the same relation to the diseases of women that *Nux* does to bilious men.

Dr. E.B. Nash

KALIUM IOD.: *Hepar Sulph.* is one of the best antidotes. Most of the reported cures with this remedy, i.e. *Kali iod.* are made with the low or crude preparations of the drug.

Dr. E.B. Nash

LYCOPODIUM: If *Lycopodium* symptomatically prescribed gives no results, give *Luesinum*, which is its best complementary.

Dr. Fergiewoods

NATRIUM SULPH.: *Sulphur* drives the patient out of bed, but *Natrum sulph.*, like *Bryonia*, is worse only after beginning to move.

Dr. E.B. Nash

SULPHUR (chronic): I think *Arsenicum* leads in all acute diseases, while *Sulphur* leads in chronic affections.

Dr. E.B. Nash

SULPHUR: *Bryonia* and *Sulphur* complement each other; but, of course, the symptoms must decide and may decide in favour of neither of them.

Dr. E.B. Nash

■

11. DIAGNOSIS THROUGH SYMPTOMS

ABORTION

Tuberculous women of the *Phosphorus* type **readily abort.**

Dr. Ellis Barker

APPENDICITIS

At all ages, any abdominal pain that has continued **without intermission** for several hours must be regarded as possible **appendicitis,** especially if it is associated with vomiting.

Dr. John Fry

ACUTE OBSTRUCTIVE APPENDICITIS

It is very **rare to find** a **clean tongue** in a case of **acute obstructive appendicitis.**

Dr. Milnes Walker

BACKACHE

To avoid backache; one rule of thumb: A woman should never lift more than 25 lbs, and a man should never lift more than half his weight.

Today's Health

BRAIN ABSCESS

Subnormal temperature, pulse and respiration with stupor, occurring in the course of a **middle ear discharge, indicates brain abscess.**

Dr. George W. Mackenzie

CANCER

Carcinoma of the rectum is a common disease and must be suspected in all patients who have persistent rectal bleeding; proctitis or procto-colitis should always be suspected when there is persistent **rectal bleeding in young people.**

Dr. Parke

The dictum *'no acid, no ulcer'* holds good in nearly all cases of peptic ulcer, and an ulcer, without free acid, suggests the presence of **Carcinoma.**

Dr. Ivy

Any irregular **bleeding from the uterus** is abnormal and must indicate a presumptive diagnosis of *Carcinoma;* this is particularly so at the climacteric.

Dr. Tomkinson

The persistence of intense **jaundice** in an old man for over 5 to 7 weeks without any other cause should be suspected as **cancer.**

Dr. S. Sen

CATARRH

Any **obstinate catarrh** that resist *Tuberculinum bovinum.*

and other remedies, should be investigated for **intestinal toxaemia** (for using bowel nosodes).

Dr. C.R. Wheeler

CERVICAL INFECTION

Lower abdominal pain, backache, and rheumatism in distant parts of the body in women, have been attributed to a cervical infection and the **cervix** has been described as the **pelvic tonsil.**

Dr. Bryan Williams

CORONARY THROMBOSIS

With an extensive coronary thrombosis, **the blood pressure may be so low that no urine is secreted** — this is a very serious symptom.

Dr. Beaumont

DIABETIC COMA

A very common observation which has been made is that, obese patients practically never develop **diabetic coma** whilst a thin, emaciated, juvenile diabetic easily develops diabetic coma.

Dr. Chari

DIABETES

Diabetes and **tuberculosis** are frequently found to exist together. Tuberculosis is far advanced, when detected in diabetic patients.

Dr. Holden

DIAGNOSIS-CHILDREN'S SICKNESS

When children are sick and show no clearly defined cause for illness, the **ears should** be invariably examined for probable infection.

Dr. H.S. Weaver

DIAGNOSIS- HEART ATTACK

Coldness of one foot, suddenly occurring after an operation, may be sign of a **"silent heart attack."**

Dr. Nathan Frank

DIAGNOSIS-CANCER

A large liver, jaundice and a normal spleen point to gall **stones or cancer;** but if the **spleen is also enlarged,** it suggests **cirrhosis of liver** or **portal obstruction.** A very enlarged spleen with, but, slightly enlarged liver suggests some of the blood diseases and needs blood examination.

Dr. S. Sen

DROPSY

Psora alone produces more marked **anasarcas** and dropsies than Sycosis; the Sycotic patient succumbs before the dropsical condition becomes marked; but the union of the two miasms produced these conditions in a marked degrees.

Dr. H.A. Roberts

EPIGASTRIC PAIN

Tuberculosis **of the spine** is the most important cause of **epigastric pain** of extra-abdominal origin. It must specially be remembered in children.

Dr. Charles Seward

EPILEPSY

In epilepsy, the remedy is not given in the actual seizure (pathological symptom) but rather in what has preceded perhaps long before.

Dr. R.O. Spalding

Abrupt loss of consciousness without faintness, sweating or palpitation, even if not preceded by any sensory aura, is almost certainly **epileptic.**

Dr. C. Kennedy

EXCESSIVE CRYING IN BABIES

A clinical examination is always necessary and particular attention should be paid **to the ears, and the urine,** since **otitis media and pyelitis** often occur silently in babies.

Dr. John Fry

GRAVE'S DISEASE

Unexplained numbness of the **chin and lower lip** must be considered an ominous indication of Grave's disease. (Carcinoma).

Dr. J.R. Calverley

HEAD INJURY

No head injury is so slight that it should be neglected, or so severe that life should be despaired of.

Dr. Bailey & Dr. Bishop

HEART DISEASE

With rare exceptions, patients with **heart disease rarely faint.**

Dr. S. Sen

INTUSSUSCEPTION

Any previously healthy child, especially between two months and two years of age, who is suddenly seized with sharp, **intermittent abdominal pain** and vomiting, should be regarded as suffering from **intussusception** and sent to hospital without delay.

Dr. Donald Court

KIDNEY DAMAGE

The appearance of **albumin** and disappearance of sugar in the urine, of a diabetic. It is an ominous sign and suggests a grave prognosis. It is an evidence of severe **kidney damage** due to the constant excretion of sugar.

Dr. Chari

LONG ILLNESS

Any child with an un-explained pallor, pyrexia, malaise or ill health of several weeks or months duration, should be suspected of having **tubercular infection.**

Dr. Balgopal Raju

MENINGITIS

The triad of severe headache, fever and vomiting should at once raise the suspicion of **Meningits,** for, in no disease is early diagnosis more important.

Dr. Charles Seward

EDEMA

Edema in the absence of dyspnoea or cardiac enlargement, is not due to heart disease.

Dr. S. Sen

ONLY TIRED

In cases without symptoms, the patient must be kept on *Sac lac,* until, you can discern some generals such as, aggravation of symptoms in the evening or at midnight.

If the patient is **only 'tired' without** guiding symptoms, you may know that it is liable to termination in some grave disorder, Tuberculosis, Bright's disease, Cancer or the like.

Dr. V.R. Carr

PARALYSIS

Causticum: Dryness of the mouth and throat; rawness of the **throat; must swallow constantly,** nervous feeling in throat. This is often a fore-runner of **paralysis.**

Dr. J.T. Kent

PATCH ON PENIS

In extravasation of urine, **a black patch on the penis** is a harbinger of death.

Dr. B. Bordie

POISONING

Dreaming of flying is an indication of **vaccinal poisoning.**

Dr. Ellis Barker

PSORA

The psoric patient is always conscious of his **heart condition** and it is he who **takes his own pulse.**

Dr. H.A. Roberts

RECURRING LUMBAGO

A history of recurring lumbago, sciatica or fibrositis, especially in young men with stiffness of back; poor chest movement and perhaps Iritis should call **Spondylitis** in mind.

Dr. Charles Seward

RETRACTED NIPPLE

In all cases of retracted nipple in young women, suspect latent **ovarian disease.**

Homeopathic Recorder

RHEUMATOID ARTHRITIS

In rheumatoid **arthritis;** the fingers and hands are stiff on **waking in the morning** and stiffness is relieved by soaking them in hot water.

In the arthritis sometimes met with in Myxoedema, (clinical syndrome of hypothyroidism) which may be mistaken for Rheumatoid Arthritis, there is no early **morning** stiffness, the patient complaining of swelling, numbness and tingling.

Dr. Beaumont

ROOT OF NAILS

Suppurative condition about the **root of the nails suggest the digestive upset** whether it is a gall bladder or liver upset or whether it is an Appendix-the patients are liable with the attack concurrently.

Dr. D.M. Borland

SLEEPING POSITIONS

Some put their **arms up above the head while sleeping.** When they sleep like that, they always have **liver disease;** always have congestion of liver. There is some trouble with liver. **But in children it is normal. In adults, it is not so.**

Dr. Piere Schmidt

STANDING STILL

It kills the psoric patients to stand still; he must walk even if he is on his feet but for a brief time; **weakness of the ankle** joints is a sure indication of the presence of combined Syphilitic and Psoric miasms.

Dr. H.A. Roberts

SUDDEN RELIEF

Always be suspicious of a **sudden cessation of symptoms** without a reaction. If the patient gets better almost instantly with no sign of a reaction, it arouses the suspicion that the action of the remedy is **only palliative.**

Dr. Boger

SYCOTIC CHILDREN

Sycotic children (so born) when one or both parents have Gonorrhoea, have cholera infantum, marasmus, pining children.

Dr. J.T. Kent

TOTALITY OF SYMPTOMS

Remember that **both subjective and objective symptoms** must enter into every case in order to make the **totality complete.**

Dr. E.B. Nash

CADMIUM: The more experience I have with the use of *Cadmium* preparations, the more convinced I am of their indispensable need in **cancer.**

Dr. A.H. Grimmer

KALIUM IOD.: The frothy expectoration is found in **oedema of the lungs** and may occur in **Bright's disease.**

Dr. E.B. Nash

LILIUM TIG.: The uterine symptoms are sometimes not marked, so as to be over-looked for the time by the violence of the **heart symptoms.**

Dr. E.B. Nash

PHOSPHORICUM ACID: It seems very singular that, after so much talk about the general depression or weakness of this remedy, we should be obliged to record that the profuse and sometimes **long-continued diarrhea should not debilitate, as a characteristic symptoms.**

Dr. E.B. Nash

STANNUM MET.: A certain physician in Albany, N.Y., was called in consultation on a **so-called case of phthisis** pulmonalis. The case was in allopathic hands. After carefully examining the case, he was asked: "what is your diagnosis, doctor?" "*Stannum met.*," said the doctor. "what! :" "*Stannum met.*," replied the doctor. *Stannum met.* was the diagnosis of the remedy, not the disease. **It was given and it cured the patient.**

Dr. E.B. Nash

∎

12. SOME REMEDIES OF SPECIFIC NATURE

CONSUMPTION

CALCAREA OSTREARUM: It is one of the most effective agents, if indicated by the **temperament and symptoms,** in the cure of this malady, and if applied at a stage when a cure is at all possible.

Dr. E.B. Nash

EPILEPSY

BUFO: We do have plenty of remedies for people who have **epilepsy.** A large percentage of the cases are curable.

Dr. J.T. Kent

FEVER

BELLADONNA: **It does not have the gradual rise** and the gradual fall, like a continued fever.

Dr. J.T. Kent

SPHERE OF MEDICINE

Every medicine has a sphere of action, a peculiar nature whereby it **differs from all other medicines** and hence it becomes suitable to complaints of one class and not suitable to those of another. It is like the **nature of human** beings, as they **differ from each other,** and also like the nature of diseases, which differ from each other in character.

Dr. J.T. Kent

STIFF NECK

BELLADONNA: It is the best remedy for **stiff neck** of rheumatic orgin or from cold.

Dr. E.A. Farrington

THIRST

BELLADONNA: It is **full of thirst,** we find it when we come to study the **stomach symptoms.**

Dr. J.T. Kent

WILL AND UNDERSTANDING

Whenever a medicine makes a man desire to do something, it affects his **will,** and when it affects his intelligence, it is acting on his **understanding.** Medicines act on both.

Dr. J.T. Kent

ACONITUM NAP.: It has two very important modalities, viz., aggravation from **fright and dry cold air.**

Dr. E.B. Nash

AETHUSA CYNAP.: (Digestion) it is at the head of the list of medicines for that condition; that is, when **digestion has absolutely ceased from brain trouble.**

Dr. J.T. Kent

ALUMINA: (Constipation) She will continue to strain, covered with **copious sweat,** hanging on to the seat, if there be any place to hang on to, and will pull and work **as if in labour,** and at last is able to expel a soft stool, yet with the sensation that more stool remains.

Dr. J.T. Kent

ANTIMONIUM CRUD.: It produces a very serious state in the mind, an **absence of the desire to live.**

Dr. J.T. Kent

ANTIMONIUM TARTARICUM: Dropsy is one of the natural conditions of all forms of *Antimonium.*

Dr. J.T. Kent

ANTIMONIUM TART.: The nausea of this remedy is as intense as that of *Ipecacuanha,* but not so persistent, and there is relief after vomiting. I have found it nearest a specific (of course we know there is no absolute specific for any disease) for cholera morbus of any remedy. For more than 25 years, I have seldom found it necessary to use any other, and then, only when there were severe cramps in the stomach and bowels, when *Cuprum metallicum* relieved.

Dr. E.B. Nash

ARGENTUM MET.: (Time) It has been an astonishing feature in this remedy that, precisely **at the hour of noon,** a great many troubles come on, and the **pains and aches; chills, headaches.**

Dr. J.T. Kent

ARGENTUM MET.: (Diabetes) It cures **albuminuria;** it cures diabetes, with **sugar in the urine;** and many of the broken down conditions of the kidneys.

Dr. J.T. Kent

ARGENTUM MET.: It is a medicine of great use in horribly **offensive leucorrhoea.** (*Kali ars., Kali phos.*)

Dr. J.T. Kent

ARGENTUM MET.: (cancer) Where it was given in, case of **scirrhus of the uterus it says,** "in less than three days, foul smell was lost entirely." When a remedy acts in that manner, it actually stops the growth. In fact, a cancerous state that would go on to its termination in 14 to 16 months will go two or three years and the patient remains comfortable. The remedy i.e. indicated, **stops the ulceration,** it checks the destruction, and keeps the patient **comfortable** and with her friends for years.

Dr. J.T. Kent

ARGENTUM NIT.: Dyspepsia, gastralgia and even **gastric ulcer** have sometimes found a powerful remedy in *Argentum nitricum,* and it has also done a great benefit in very obstinate **cases of diarrhea of various kinds.**

Dr. E.B. Nash

ARNICA MONT.: I have often relieved sewing girls or students, of **pains in the eyes** from this cause and have sometimes enabled them to lay off the glasses that had been prescribed by the opticians. It is much better to use this remedy in a **weakened power of accommodation** than to try and compensate for it with artificial lenses. Of course, where the **impaired vision is purely optical, this cannot be done.**

Dr. E.B. Nash

ARSENICUM ALBUM: *Arsenic* and *Merc-corr.* are the two principal medicines for **spreading ulcerations** which eat in every direction and the discharges are very offensive.

Dr. J.T. Kent

ARSENICUM ALB.: (Stomach and skin) I once had a case of very severe **gastralgia caused by suppression of eczema** on the hands. I knew nothing of the suppression, but prescribed *Arsenicum* because, the pains came on at midnight, lasting until 3 A.M., during which time the patient had to walk the floor in agony, and there was great burning in the stomach. She had, but one slight attack after taking *Arsenicum*, but, said she, when I visited her, "doctor, would that remedy send out salt rheum?." Then I found out about the suppression which had been caused by the application of an ointment, and told her that she could have back the pain in the stomach any time she wanted it, by suppressing the eruption again. She did not want it.

Dr. E.B. Nash

ARSENICUM ALB.: (Asthma) It is particularly efficacious in many affections of the lungs, where the **breathing is very much oppressed. Respiration is wheezing,** with cough and frothy expectoration . Patient cannot lie down, must sit up to breathe, and is unable to move without being greatly put out of breath. **The air passages seem constricted.** It is especially useful in asthmatic affections caused or aggravated by suppressed eruptions, like pneumonia from retrocedent measles, or **even chronic lung troubles from suppressed eczema.**

Dr. E.B. Nash

ASAFOETIDA: (Asthma) **Asthmatic attacks at least once a day all her life,** brought on by every bodily exertion, coition and especially **by every satisfying meal.**

Dr. J.T. Kent

ASAFOETIDA: I never like to see them come into my office, for they are **hard cases to manage.**

Dr. J.T. Kent

AURUM MET.: *Aurum met.* is one of the few remedies that has hemiopia or half-sightedness and has cured it even in the 200th potency. *Lycopodium* and *Lithium carbonicum* also have half-sightedness, but **Aurum sees only the lower,** while the other **two see only the left half of objects.**

Dr. E.B. Nash

AURUM MET. : I once cured a young lady who tried to **commit suicide by drowning.** After she was cured she laughed at the occurrence, and said she could not help it. It seemed to her she was of no use in the world. She felt so.

Dr. E.B. Nash

AURUM MET.: You **take away a man's hope** and he has nothing to live for, he then wants to die. Such, it seems, is the state in this medicine.

Dr. J.T. Kent

BELLADONNA: (Boil) It is astonishing how many local inflammations, even a carbuncle or **boil,** will so disturb the general system and circulation, as to produce the general inflammatory fever, with the characteristic head symptoms calling for *Belladonna,* and no less astonishing is, how this remedy controls the whole condition, both local and general, when indicated. What! exclaims the believer in local applications, give *Belladonna* internally for a boil on the hand or foot? Yes, indeed, not only *Belladonna*, but *Mercurius, Hepar sulphuris, Tarantula cubensis,* and many others, and **you will not have any need for local medication at all.**

Dr. E.B. Nash

CALCAREA CARB.: An **opacity itself,** when it is present, is not a symptom, **but a result of disease.**

Dr. J.T. Kent

CALCAREA CARB: (Suffocation) The *Calcarea* patient **can't go upstairs;** he is so tired in his legs, and so tired in the chest; he pants and **suffocates from going upstairs.** He has every evidence of muscular weakness and flabbiness. Nutrition is impaired everywhere. This is the kind of patient that used to be called **scrofulous;** now we call the condition **psora;** and *Calcarea* in one of our deepest anti-psoric. It is a medicine that goes deep into the life, and takes a deep hold of every part of the economy.

Dr. J.T. Kent

CALCAREA CARB: (Confusion) Any amount of **thinking becomes impossible.** It is almost impossible for him to come to a conclusion, for he never figures it twice alike.

Dr. J.T. Kent

CALCAREA CARB: (Loathes life) When an individual ceases to love his own life, and is weary of it, and loathes it, and wants to die, he is on the border line of insanity. In fact, that is **an insanity of the will,** you have only to look with an observing eye, to, see that one may be **insane in the**

affections, or **insane in the intelligence.** One may remain quite intact, and the other one be destroyed.

Dr. J.T. Kent

CALCAREA CARB.: (Hair fall) **The hair fall out,** not in the regular way such as occurs in old age, but in **patches here and there.**

Dr. J.T. Kent

CALCAREA CARB.: (Internal heat - external cold) It is a peculiar feature of *Calcarea* that, the more marked the **congestion of internal parts, the colder** the surface becomes. With chest troubles, and stomach troubles, and bowel troubles, **the feet and hands become like ice, and covered with sweat;** and he lies in bed sometimes with a fever in the rest of his body, and the **scalp covered with cold sweat.**

Dr. J.T. Kent

CALCAREA OST.: We must not omit to notice the action of *Calcarea ost.* on the **respiratory organs,** for the reason that it is of great importance in its use in that dreaded disease, **pulmonary consumption.**

Dr. E.B. Nash

CARBO VEG.: No true remark was ever written that *Carbo veg.* is especially adapted to cachectic individuals whose **vital powers have become weakened.** This remark is made particularly clear when considered in the light of those cases in which disease seems to be **engrafted upon the system** by reason of the depressing influence of some prior derangement.

Dr. Henry N. Guernsey

CARBO VEG · (Last stage) Of course, no remedy can raise the dead, no matter how strong the indications before death; **but no remedy can come nearer than this** and the dominant school knows little or nothing about it, and never can, until they will consent to use it in the homeopathic form and according to homeopathic indications.

Dr. E.B. Nash

CAULOPHYLLUM: I have given this remedy in long continued **passive haemorrhage** from the uterus after miscarriage, when I had the characteristic weakness and sense of **internal trembling present in the patient.**

Dr. E.B. Nash

CHAMOMILLA: (Irritable) There is a remedy for inflammation of the **tonsils where the ear** is envolved and is ameliorated by heat, but very few use it, it is of great value; it is *Chamomilla*, and it is especially indicated if the **patient is irritable.**

Dr. J.T. Kent

CICUTA VIR.: It is also a good remedy for the effects of **concussion of the brain or spine,** if spasms are in the train of chronic effects therefrom and *Arnica* **does not relieve.**

Dr. E.B. Nash

CUPRUM: Tones down, **relieves that sensitivity,** and well **selected remedies** will then act curatively.

Dr. J.T. Kent

DIGITALIS PUR.: (Jaundice) A young man of good habits was taken with nausea and vomiting. He was **drowsy,** and after a couple of days he began to **grow very pale and**

chlorotic all over. The sclerotica were as yellow as gold, as was, indeed, the skin all over the body, even **to the nails.** The stools were natural as to consistence, but **perfectly colourless,** while the urine was as brown as lager beer, or even more so. Where you could see through it, on the edge of the receptacle, it was **yellow as fresh bile.** The **pulse was only thirty beats per minute,** and often dropped out a beat.

This was a perfect *Digitalis* case of **jaundice,** and this remedy cured him perfectly in a few days, improvement in his feelings taking place very shortly after beginning it; the stools, urine and skin gradually taking on their natural colour. The **characteristic slow pulse was the leading** symptoms to the prescription, for all the rest of the symptoms may be found in almost any well-developed case of severe jaundice.

Dr. E.B. Nash

HELONIAS DIO.: (Anaemia) There is almost always associated with it a more or less anaemic condition. This anaemia may seem to be consequent upon, **too profuse menstruation** or flooding, or it may exist entirely independent of any such cause. In these cases, I have often found **albumen present in the urine,** sometimes in large quantities, especially in **pregnant women,** and see rapid improvement and disappearance of the albumen under the action of this remedy.

Dr. E.B. Nash

HYOSCYAMUS NIG.: If acute delirium passes on into **the settled form, called mania,** this remedy is still one of our chief reliances.

Dr. E.B. Nash

HYOSCYAMUS NIG: "Every muscle in the body twitches, from the eyes to the toes." This is one of its chief indications for its use in convulsions, whether epileptic or not.

Dr. E.B. Nash

IPECACUANHA: (Anaemic) It is true that, when patients have bled, until they have become anaemic, and are subject to dropsy, *Ipecacuanha* to be the remedy; its **natural follower then is China**, which will bring the patient in a position to need an anti-psoric remedy.

Dr. J.T. Kent

KALIUM IOD.: (pneumonia) '*Kali iod.*' in the words of E.A. Farrington, "pneumonia, in which disease, it is an excellent remedy **when hepatization has commenced,** when the disease localizes itself, and infiltration begins. In such cases, in the **absence of other symptoms calling distinctively for** *Bryonia, Phosphorus* or *Sulphur*, I would advise you to select *Iodine* or *Iodide* of potass. It is also called for, when the hepatization is so extensive that we have **cerebral congestion,** or even an effusion into the brain as a result of this congestion.

Dr. E.B. Nash

LACHESIS: (Climacteric) In short, the **circulation** in *Lachesis* subjects is **very uncertain.** This is what makes it so valuable in sudden **flushes during the climacteric period.**

Dr.,E.B. Nash

LYCOPODIUM: A feeling of **satiety** is found under this remedy which alternates with a **feeling of hunger** of a peculiar kind.

Dr. E.B. Nash

NATRIUM MUR.: (Anaemia) **It is one of our best remedies for anaemia. It does not seem to make much difference** whether the anaemia is caused by **loss of fluids**(*China, Kali carb.*), **menstrual irregularities** (*Puls.*), **loss of semen** (*Phos. acid, China*), grief or other mental diseases.

Dr. E.B. Nash

NATRIUM MUR.: Headache is apt to occur after the menstrual period, as if caused by **loss of blood,** and you know that *China* also has throbbing headache in such cases. with *Natrums,* **the throbbing headache occurs whether the menses be scanty or profuse.**

Dr. E.B. Nash

OPIUM & GLONOINUM: They equalize the circulation, and the patient may not die.

Dr. J.T. Kent

PODOPHYLLUM: (Jaundice) I once made a brilliant cure of an **obstinate case of intermittent** fever with this remedy. The chills were very violent and were followed by intense fever with great loquacity. There was also **great jaundice present.**

Dr. E.B. Nash

PODOPHYLUM: If you had a child with copious, gushing, violently foetid stool, **ameliorated by lying on the abdomen,** and it would have another stool if lying any other way, *Podophyllum* would be the remedy.

Dr. J.T. Kent

SABADILLA: A sleepiness comes on from thinking, meditating, reading. While meditating in a chair, **he falls**

asleep like *Nux moschata* and *Phosphoric acid.*

Dr. J.T. Kent

SECALE COR.: I have never, in a practice of 35 years, used it in this way, but have always been able to **control such haemorrhages.** *Secale cor.* is not often indicated in active post-partum haemorrhages.

Dr. E.B. Nash

SILICEA: It does not increase in size or strength, learns to **walk late;** in short, if not actually sick in bed, everything seems to have **come to standstill so far as growth or development is concerned.**

Dr. E.B. Nash

SILICEA: It is the remedy to restore and **cure such sweats,** by correcting the **conditions upon which the sweat depend.**

Dr. E.B. Nash

SPONGIA TOST.: The dry, chronic, sympathetic **cough** of **organic heart disease** is oftener and more permanently relieved by this remedy **than by** *Naja.* *Spongia* is also a **good remedy for goitre,** with sense of suffocation after sleep.

Dr. E.B. Nash

SULPHUR: Let no one understand that *Sulphur* is the only remedy capable of removing **psoric complications,** but simply that, *Sulphur* will be likely to be **oftener indicated** here, because it oftener covers the usual manifestations of psora in its pathogenesis than any other remedy. There are anti-psorics, like *Psorinum, Causticum, Graphites,* etc., which may have to be used instead of *Sulphur* and we know which one, by the same law which guides us in the selection of the right remedy and time.

Dr. E.B. Nash

SULPHUR: No one need tell me that there is no relation of skin to internal troubles. I have seen too much of it, and have cured many cases of that character, **where a restoration of the skin disease relieved the internal** trouble which had followed its retrocession or suppression.

Dr. E.B. Nash

■

KING AND CAUTION

Crataegus is believed to be he king of heart tonics.

Dr. T.M. Moore

The drug may cause nausea when given in the tincture unless given during or immediately after meals, thus nausea with weakness may be a leading indication

Dr. J.H. Clarke

Acts on muscle of heart, and is a heart tonic. Must be used for some time in order to obtain good results.

Dr. Wm. Boericke.

13. POTENCIES

BACKACHE

Gelsemium should never be forgotten in inveterate backache. It is recommended in doses all the way from 10 drops of Q to 10M.

Medical century, 1893

CORNS

In addition to *Antimonium crudum* for corns in general, recent or painful corns, *Ferrum pic.* 3 is useful and very effective, and for the constitutional tendency, *Radium brom.* 30 once a fortnight will give the patient a new lease of life.

Dr. Pettitt

CHANGE OF REMEDY

Never change a remedy that has done good, **until** you have given it in a higher potency.

Dr. Hughes

FEVER BLISTERS

Some 80% of fever blisters can be quickly cured often in 36 hours with *Natrum mur.* in 6x, 12x or 30th potencies. I have seen some cases of fever blisters cured as if from magic with *Rananculus bulb.*, or *Rananculus-s.*, which would not respond to *Natrum mur.* in any potency.

Dr. E. Petrie Hoyle

HIGH POTENCIES

It is well for you to realize that you are **dealing with razors** when dealing with **high potencies.** I would rather be in the room with a **dozen negroes slashing with razors** than in the hands of an ignorant prescriber of high potencies. They are means of tremendous **harm as well as of tremendous good.**

Dr. J.T. Kent

PATHOLOGICAL PRESCRIBING

One may prescribe on a pathological basis where a remedy is known to have a relationship with certain tissues, for e.g. *Hepar sulph.* for suppuration, *Silicea* for inflammation near bone, *Bryonia* for serous tissues. **The potency in pathological** prescribing is important, for if the patient's vitality is low, **a high potency may make too big demands on the system** and harm rather than doing good.

Dr. Grace H. Newell

POTENCIES

Acute cases

In **high temperatures, use the medium potency i.e. 200**[th] and repeat night and morning until reaction occurs.

Dr. Boger

Hypersensitive patients

For **hyper sensitive patients,** use low or medium potencies.

Dr. Stuart Clouse

Incurable cases

High potencies will not **palliate incurable cases;** you must use **the low.**

Dr. Boger

You do not build mole hills out of our high potencies; they **simply establish a state of order,** so that digestion and assimilation go on, order is established and the tissues are improved. Health comes, beauty, growth of hair, better skin and better nails.

Dr. J.T. Kent

POTENCY

When reaction is delayed in distressing crisis after a potency as low as the 200th or 1m has been given, go to the 50m or higher and grateful relief will ensue.

Dr. R.E.S. Hayes

THREE DOSES

In acute conditions, **never give more than three doses of a remedy in the same potency.** If patient is much better or worse after any one dose, do not repeat. Later it may be necessary to repeat the **remedy in a higher potency.**

Homeo. Recorder, June 28

ANTIMONIUM TART.: If *Sulphur* is not able to promote **absorption** in a case, *Tartar emetic* will often do it. I have used it from the **200th to the cm. potencties** with equally good results.

Dr. E.B. Nash

ARGENTUM NITR.: Allen and Norton write as follows: " the greatest service that *Argentum nitricum* performs is in **purulent ophthalmia.** With large experience, in both — hospitals and private practice, we have not lost a single eye from this disease, and every one has been treated with internal remedies, most of them with *Argentum nitricum* of a **high potency, 30th or 200th.**

Dr. E.B. Nash

AURUM MET.: *Aurum met.* is one of the few remedies that has hemiopia or **half-sightedness,** and has cured it **even in the 200th** potency.

Dr. E.B. Nash

BACILLINUM: I use *Bacillinum* 30 in incipient **tuberculosis.** In early cases, it is my custom to give a dose, once every 10 days to two weeks. I have had many early cases that cleared up after a few months treatment with this preparation. **In late stage of tuberculosis,** Bacillinum is of no benefit.

Dr. Walter sands mills

BAPTISIA TINCT.: We have repeatedly proved its value in fevers apparently simple, but which **failed to yield to Aconite.** It should be given in a low dilution, 1x, or even the strong tincture.

Dr. Ruddock

BAPTISIA TINCT.: I have used both, the low and high preparations with equal success, but now use the 30th potency.

Dr. E.B. Nash

BENZOIC AC.: Ganglions were dispersed by *Benzoic acid* given internally in the dilutions from the 12th and the 30th potency.

Dr. Turrel

CAMPHORA OFF.: (Collapse) *Camphor* is the first remedy to be thought of, and according to susceptibility or strength of the patient, the dose must be varied from **tincture to highest potency.**

Dr. E.B. Nash

CANNABIS SAT.: I used them **all in the cm.**, and I know, having tried both, that **they cure better than the low potencies.**

Dr. E.B. Nash

CANNABIS SATIVA.: I used in my **early practice** to put five drops mother tincture into four ounces of water (in a four ounce vial) and let the patient take a teaspoonful three times a day. After about four days the inflammatory symptoms would have subsided, and the thin discharge have thickened and become greenish in appearance. Then *Mercurius sol.* 3d trituration, a powder three times a day, would often finish the case. Or if a little, thin, gleety discharge remained, I cured that with *Sulphur, Capsicum* or Kali iod.. I have cured many cases in, from one to two weeks, this way. **Later I have used the c.m. poteny in the first stage, and sometimes never have to use the second remedy.**

Dr. E.B. Nash

CAULOPHYLLUM: I advise to try *Caulophyllum* in high potency. I did so in the **200th potency** and cured the whole case promptly and permanently.

Dr. E.B. Nash

CICUTA VIR.: I once had a case of **eczema capitis** in a young woman. It was of long standing and covered the whole scalp, solid, like a cap. I gave her *Cicuta* 200th and cured her completely in a very short time.

Dr. E.B. Nash

CINCHONA OFF.: *China* will do excellent service. It is equally good in **splenic diseases** which closely resemble the splenic troubles resulting from the abuse of quinine. I have found the **200th do better than lower potencies.**

Dr. E.B. Nash

COFFEA CRUD.: Coffea has won to itself great credit as a **sleep remedy.** In my experience and observation, it works best **here in the 200th potency.**

Dr. E.B. Nash

GELSEMIUM SEMP.: I consider the **large doses** of either (Opium and Gels.) remedy used by some to quiet excited conditions, or to control **spasms or convulsions** by their toxic, depressing, or paralyzing action on the muscular system, antipathic, and in no way truly curative. I have never known the remedy to do much good in these conditions below **the 30th potency,** but often in the **potencies much above that.**

Dr. E.B. Nash

HAMAMELIS VIR.: In **varicose veins** of the leg, you will be delighted with the way in which the first or second dilution of *Hamamelis* will cure the pain.

Dr. Hughes

IGNATIA AMARA: In one case of puerperal **convulsions,** other remedies having failed to do any good, the consulting physician while observing the patient during one of the spasms, noticed that she came out of it with a succession of **long drawn sighs.** He inquired if the patient had any recent mental trouble, and learned that she had **lost her mother, of whom she was exceedingly fond,** and whom she had mourned for greatly, a few weeks before. *Ignatia* 30th quickly cured her.

Dr. E.B. Nash

IODIUM: I have cured many cases of **goitre with** *Iodium* **C.M. poency,** when indicated, giving a powder every night for four nights, after the **moon fulled and was waning.**

Dr. E.B. Nash

IPECACUANHA: It is a better remedy than *Secale cor.*, ever was or can be, for **post-partum haemorrhages,** and it is not necessary to use it in large and poisonous doses, for it will stop them in the **200th potency,** and is quicker in its action than *Secale.*

Dr. E.B. Nash

IRIS VERS.: I used to give the remedy in the 3d; but of late years have given it in the **50m.** and I am better pleased with the result, because it is **more prompt and lasting.**

Dr. E.B. Nash

KALIUM BICH.: I have with it cured many cases of **diphtheritic croup,** and of late years never given it below the 30th **potency,** because, abundant experience has convinced me that it does better than the low triturations.

Dr. E.B. Nash

KALIUM CARB.: (Potency) If you give *Kali-carb*, to one of the **incurable patients in very high potency, it will make your patient worse,** and the aggravation will be serious and prolonged, but the **30th potency may be of great service.**

Dr. J.T. Kent

KALIUM IOD.: I used to dissolve two to four grains of the crude salt in a four ounce vial of water and direct the patient to take a teaspoonful of this preparation three times a day, until it is half used, and then fill up with water and continue taking the same way until cured; filling up the vial every time of this description and feeling sure of my remedy, I **gave it in the 200th potency as an experiment.** This case also made fully as speedy a recovery as the others treated with the crude drug, so since then I often prescribe it in the potencies.

Dr. E.B. Nash

KALIUM IOD.: I think it can be **used lower than most drugs without injury,** and yet I believe we do not know half its remedial power as developed by our process of potentisation.

Dr. E.B. Nash

KREOSOTUM: (vomit) I have used it here also in the 200th. *Kreosote* is also one of our best remedies in other kinds of vomiting; in the **vomiting of pregnancy** and in that other intractable disease of the stomach, known as **gastromalacia.**

Dr. E.B. Nash

KREOSOTUM: One has seen *Kreosote* 200 annihilative of the terrible odours that sometimes accompany **cancer of the cervix,** where, if it did nothing more, it made life more supportable for patient and for entourage.

Dr. M.L. Tyler

LAC CAN.: *Lac caninum* cured the case very quickly, not long after I had a very severe case of scarlatina. The throat was swollen full, and restlessness was so marked with pains in the limbs which left the patient tossing from side to side that **I thought surely** *Rhus tox.* **must be the remedy. But it failed to relieve.** Then I discovered that the soreness of the throat and the **pains alternated sides.** This called to my mind the remedy, which was given with prompt relief. **I used the cm. in this case.**

Dr. E.B. Nash

NATRIUM MUR.: (Potency) Isn't it curious how some physicians will hoot at a potency and fly like a frightened crow from a bacillus varying in size from 0.004 m.m. to 0.006m.m. They can hardly eat, drink or sleep for the fear that a little microbe of the fifteenth culture will light on them somewhere, but there is nothing in a potency above the 12th. **When prejudice gives way to honest, earnest investigation for truth,** the world may be better for it.

Dr. E.B. Nash

PODOPHYLLUM PELT.: In the first onset of the disease, as well as in the very far advanced and apparently hopeless cases of **cholera infantum,** the 100th potency (B. &T.) has done the best for me.

Dr. E.B. Nash

PULSATILLA: Don't pour down mother tincture of *Pulsatilla* by the 10 drop doses, as is the manner of those who do not believe in potentized remedies. You may give

Pulsatilla in the high, higher, and highest potencies, and confidently expect the best results. I have often seen the **delayed menses of young girls** of *Pulsatilla* temperament appear promptly and naturally **under the mm. of swan and cm. of fincke** (also with *Kali carbonicum, Tuberculinum),* and other).

Dr. E.B. Nash

RHUS TOX.: (Potency) I have used it both high and low, and found it useful all along the scale, but **I have m.m. potency** made upon my own potentizer which has served me so well, and so many times, that I cannot refrain from speaking of it.

Dr. E.B. Nash

SARSAPARILLA OFF.: *Sarsaparilla* is one of the best remedies for **headache or periosteal pains** generally, from suppressed gonorrhoea. I have seen great results from the **200th potency.**

Dr. E.B. Nash

SECALE COR.: All the **toes were attacked** with **dry gangrene.** A few doses of *Secale cor.* (high), afforded great relief, and checked the progress of the disease for a long time.

Dr. E.B. Nash

SELENIUM MET.: **Bad effects from drinking too much tea;** all complaints are aggravated by it. **Irresistible longing** for spirituous liquors. Hoarseness, must often clear the throat of mucus, especially at the beginning of singing. Irresistible desire for stimulants, wants to get drunk but feels worse after

after It. Very forgetful. I have never used this metal below 200th potency.

Dr. E.B. Nash

SPONGIA TOSTA: I live in a **croupy** climate and district, and after experimenting for 30 years, first with the low, then with the higher preparations, affirm that the **200th potency** of this remedy does **better work in croup** than the lower preparations.

Dr. E.B. Nash

STRAMONIUM: I cured a case just as bad since then, with the cm. potency.

Dr. E.B. Nash

SULPHUR: In cm. potency—it is generally efficacious in the case of **ganglion.**

Dr. J.H. Clarke

SULPHUR: Those who use the potentized *Sulphur*, **can ever know what it is capable of curing.**

Dr. E.B. Nash

SYPHILINUM: It is a cure for **caries of the spine** of long standing by *Syphilinum* (high). I had a very similar case, for which I had been prescribing **for over a year without success,** when I first read the report of this case. In my case, as in his, the patient had severe pains in the diseased part **during the night.** Every one acquinted with syphilitic troubles, especially of the bones, knows of these (terrible, sometimes) nightly bone pains. Three doses of **Swan's** *Syphilinum* **cm. cured this case in the remarkably short space of 40 days.**

Dr. E.B. Nash

THYROIOD: The use of *Thyroidin.* in 30 or 200 dilution will not only **prevent grey hair** but help in restoring natural colour. Give 30 for one month daily thereafter 200 every week for one month.

Dr. R.B. Das

■

CAUSE OF GENERAL DECLINE IN HEALTH

We can see a trend of general decline in health of the people. The cause in Two-fold — fear and tension' in life. Our aspirations have gone too high - and the fear of failure has increased. Constant tension is disturbing the normal function of the organs and there by - the whole body and its system.

Other causes become secondary fact above two factors.

14. GENERAL

ANTIDOTES

All substances consumed as food become great remedies, such as vinegar, coffee, common salt, etc. We should look to them oftener than we do for the stubborn chronic cases.

Dr. J.T. Kent

APPEARANCE

Experienced physicians **learn to classify** patients by appearance.

Dr. J.T. Kent

APPETIZER

Cinchona rubra and *Gentian* Q in combination, 10 drops to be taken before meals, is an appetizer.

Dr. Ellis Barker

BILIARY COLIC

In biliary colic, *Calcarea carb.* has **never failed** me.

Dr. Hughes

BURNS

For burns by stove or matches, **quick douche** in cold water seems to promote faster pain relief and faster healing.

Dr. King

CAUTIONS

You do not get the full benefit of homeopathy and you **cannot stop his stimulants because weakness will follow.** Persons who have not taken wine as a regular beverage can and should do without it, as it interferes with the action of the homeopathic remedy.

Dr. J.T. Kent

CLOSE OBSERVATION

You do not get all these things in the text, you have to see them applied, but the things I give you, that are brought out clinically, are those things that have come from applying the symptoms of the remedy at the bed side to sick folks.

Dr. J.T. Kent

CONSCIENCIOUS PHYSICIAN

It is quite a profitable business for one who has not much conscience and not much intelligence. But conscientious physician feels worried and knows he is not doing what he ought to do with his patient, unless he reaches out for the remedy which touches the constitution. **It is far more useful to keep people from taking colds than to cure colds.**

Dr. J.T. Kent

CONSTIPATION

A glass of cold water, on rising in the morning, with a level teaspoon of common table salt makes an excellent **laxative.**

Dr. Wheeler.

DIABETES

Syzygium Q and *Uranium nit.*3x both combined or one after the other t.d.s. **reduce the sugar** in the urine in a fort-night.

Dr. Ghosal

HOMEOPATHIC FAILURES

The homeopathic failures are the **worst failures on earth.**

Dr. J.T. Kent

INSOMNIA

It is seldom that the drug homeopathically choosen fails to relieve insomnia. If there are no clear indications, *Passiflora* Q and *Avena sat.* Q in doses from 3 to 5 or more drops are useful aids and **do not establish any drug habit.**

Dr. Ruddock

LAME THERAPEUTICS

Now-a-days, **washing out** the stomach by lavage, and the rectum and colon by enemas, according to *"hall's method,"* is quite fashionable, and is withal much more sensible, in as much as they are so lame in their therapeutics.

Dr. E.B. Nash

MIASMS

Finally don't forget to look for the **three miasms** in all **obstinate cases,** whether acute or chronic.

Dr. E.B. Nash

NASH-TISSUE REMEDIES

I have **no faith** in the Schuesslerian theory in regard to it. Similia Similibus Curantur has stood the test with other remedies, and will, with the **so called tissues** remedies, regardless of theories.

Dr. E.B. Nash

NATURE PROVIDES FOR THE REGION

Another idea has been advanced that, in any particular region, the **vegetable kingdom** provides all that is necessary for curing in that region.

Dr. J.T. Kent

OBEDIENCE TO TRUTH

We owe **no obedience to man,** not even to our parents, after we are old enough to think for ourselves. We owe obedience to truth.

Dr. J.T. Kent

REPETITION

You can **never definitely determine** the power of the potentised remedy, but you should be able to realize when it is exhausted and its further application futile.

Dr. Boger

RHEUMATISM

Inter-costal rheumatism **yields far more quickly** to *Rananculus bulb.* than to any other. (*Aconite, Arnica, Bryonia.*)

Dr. E.A. Farrington

SELECTION OF A REMEDY

No remedy should ever be given on one symptom. If you are led to a remedy by a peculiar symptom, study the remedy and the disease thoroughly to ascertain, if the two are similar enough to each other, to expect a cure. Any deviation from that rule is ruinous and will lead to the practice of giving medicines on single symptom.

Dr. J.T. Kent

Partly Indicated Remedies

Remedies only partly related to the case **will change the character** of the sickness so that no one can cure the case.

Dr. J.T. Kent

Nature of the Case

Be sure that the remedy has not only the group of symptoms, but also the nature of the case.

Dr. J.T. Kent

SELF CLEANING SYSTEM

Notwithstanding these improvements, there is still a great deal of "gut scraping" going on in the name of "cleaning out the system," **as though** the alimentary canal was not a self-cleaning institution, if kept, or put into a healthy condition, but must be regularly "gone through" once in about so often, on the **"house cleaning" principle.**

Dr. E.B. Nash

SLEEPLESSNESS

For the production of sleep, no remedy compares with *Hyoscyamus* in tincture 5 to 10 drops in half a glass of water and teaspoonful doses given half hourly.

Dr. Butler

STUDY OF PATIENT

Hering's advice when he says "treat the patient, not the disease."

Dr. E.B. Nash

SUCCESSFUL CURE

Prescribe for the patient first. **No results of disease should be removed until** proper constitutional treatment has been restored to, and be sure that it is proper.

Dr. J.T. Kent

SYMPTOMS

Examine every organ, not by examining it physically, for **results of diseases do not lead to the remedy,** but examine the symptoms.

Dr. J.T. Kent

THREE KINGDOMS

There seems to be everything existing in one kingdom that exists in another. Then lowest is the **mineral,** the next the **vegetable,** and last the **animal kingdom.** If we had a perfect knowledge of any one of the kingdom, we could probably cover the entire scope of curative possibilities. But

we have only a knowledge of a few remedies in each
kingdom.

Dr. J.T. Kent

WOUNDS

The sides of a cut must be drawn together, and if it is
perfectly tight, it will heal itself by first intention. **If it does
not**, then you may know there is a constitutional condition
that you must find out and find the remedy for it. Local
treatment must then be suspended. These remedies, that I
have mentioned, to a great extent, cover the management **if
wounds are simple.** Anyone has sense enough to draw
together and close up a yawning wound, and to properly
dress it. The muscles that naturally draw a wound open
have to be overcome by stitching or by strappings. They do
not belong to prescribing, **they belong to the surgeon.**

Dr. J.T. Kent

Air is an irritant to a raw part and will keep up an
unnecessary discharge of pus, even from a perfectly healthy
sore.

Dr. J.T. Kent

REMEDIES

ACONITUM NAP.: It is very seldom that fear will give
a man inflammation, **but fear is a common** cause of
inflammation of the uterus, and of the ovaries, in plethoric,
vigorous, excitable woman.

Dr. J.T. Kent

ALLIUM CEPA: For the **neuralgic pains (after operation on the eye)** which often occur within the first 24 hours, relief can frequently be obtained from **5 drop doses of the tincture** of *Allium cepa*.

Dr. Norton

ANTIMONIUM TART.: With Tartar emetic the, **face is always pale,** or cyanotic, with no redness, and the breathing is not stertorous.

Dr. E.B. Nash

ANTIMONIUM TART.: It is also one of our best remedies for **hepatization of lungs remaining after pneumonia.** There is dullness on percussion, and lack, or absence of respiratory murmur, and shortness of breath, and patient continues to be pale, weak and sleepy.

Dr. E.B. Nash

ARGENTUM NIT.: (Conjunctivitis) "I do believe that there is no need of cauterization with it, except in the gonorrheal form of purulent conjunctivitis." Such testimony from such sources, ought to shame the abuse of this agent in the hands of old school physicians, and sometimes **bogus homeopaths. In ophthalmia neonatorum,** in my own practice as a general practitioner, I have had very often **better success** with **Mercurius solubilis,** especially where there was much purulent matter pouring out on opening the eyes.

Dr. A.B. Norton

BAPTISIA TINCT.: Typhoid fever can be aborted under proper homeopathic treatment, no matter what the old school says to the contrary.

Dr. E.B. Nash

BELLIS PER.. It is a grand friend to commercial travellers and **railway spine of moderate severity,** it has no substitute, so far as my knowledge reaches. I think stasis lies at the bottom of these ailings.

Dr. Burnett

BENZOICUM AC.: Both *Benzoicum acid* and *Berberis vul.* are great remedies for **arthritic troubles with the urinary symptoms.**

Dr. E.B. Nash

BENZOICUM AC.: In dribbling of urine of old men with enlarge prostate, it has done good service. The urine in the clothing **scents the whole room.**

Dr. E.B. Nash

BISMUTHUM: It is also often of **benefit in cancer of the stomach,** when there is at times vomiting of enormous quantities of food that seems to **have lain in the stomach for days.**

Dr. E.B. Nash

BORAX VEN.: It has also white, albuminous, starchy leucorrhoea, quite profuse, and with a **sensation of warm water running down.**

Dr. E.B. Nash

CALCAREA PHOS.: Diarrhea is very prominent, and the stools are green and **"spluttering",** that is, the flatulence (of which there is much) with the stool makes a loud **spluttering noise** when the stool passes.

Dr. E.B. Nash

CAUSTICUM: *Causticum* has all grades of nervous twitchings, chorea, **convulsions and epileptic attacks,** even progressive **locomotor ataxia.**

Dr. E.B. Nash

CAUSTICUM: Painful stiffness of the back and sacrum, especially on rising from a chair.

Dr. E.B. Nash

CHAMOMILLA: We might draw lines of differentiation between this and other **restless remedies,** but it would take too long. Each physician must get a habit of doing this for himself. In his ability to do this, lies the superior skilfulness of the homeopathic practitioner.

Dr. E.B. Nash

DIOSCOREA VILL.: 15 drops of tincture in hot water will cause the intense pain of **appendicitis** to fade away and give ease to the patient.

Dr. Anchutz

GELSEMIUM SEMP.: One author says that *Gelsemium* stands **midway** between *Aconite* and *Veratrum viride*. I should rather place it **between** *Baptisia* and *Belladonna*.

Dr. E.B. Nash

GELSEMIUM SEMP.: It is useful in the remittent fever of children. The fever is never of that active or violent form calling for *Aconite* or *Belladonna*, but of a **milder form.** The child lies drowsy, does not want to move, or, if it does, cannot move much on account of the weakness.

Dr. E.B. Nash

KALI CARB.: (Chronic of Colocynth) There are plenty of short acting remedies that would relieve the pain speedily, and at the close of the attack the constitutional remedy could then be given. If the patient can bear the pain to the end, it is better to wait until it passes off without any medicine. That sometimes is cruel, and then, the short acting medicines should be given.

Dr. J.T. Kent

KALMIA LAT.: (Heart and kidney) All the organs are related to each other, but especially the heart and kidneys. When the kidneys are not working well, the heart is very often troublesome. All through the varying forms of Bright's disease, the heart is troublesome. Difficulties of breathing, difficult heart action, with albuminuria. It will relieve the breathing. Again, associated with kidney affections, we have many eye complaints, difficulties of vision, and these also especially call for this remedy. It is often indicated in Bright's disease, with disturbance of vision, occurring during pregnancy.

Dr. J.T. Kent

KREOSOTUM: (Cancer of uterus) The case with the lochia after confinement, when the choice may lie between these three remedies, *Kreosote, Rhus tox.* and *Sulphur.* The other symptoms must decide between them. This ulceration may be found in cancer of the uterus, and then *Kreosote* will often be of great value. I have no doubt that, many cases which degenerate into cancer, might be prevented by its timely use. In some cases there is awful burning in the pelvis, as of red-hot coals, with discharge of clots in foul smelling blood. I see that *Guernsey* recommends it in cancer of the mammae, saying it is hard, bluish-red and covered with scurvy protuberances. I have never so used it, but in **corrosive leucorrhoeas and ulcerations,** I have and with great satisfaction. I generally use it in the 200th, with simply tepid water injections for cleanliness.

Dr. J.T. Kent

LACHESIS: It is **seldom** that you will see *Lachesis* **headaches without cardiac difficulty.**

Dr. J.T. Kent

LACHESIS: The symptoms of *Lachesis* have sometimes to be taken years after.

Dr. J.T. Kent

MEDORRHINUM: (Time) The most characteristic difference between them is that, with *Medorrhinum,* the pains are worse in **the day-time,** and with *Syphilinum* **in the night.**

Dr. E.B. Nash

MURIATICUM AC.: (Typhoid) There is **decomposition of fluids;** the stools are involuntary while passing urine; stools dark, thin, or haemorrhage of dark liquid blood. Mouth full of dark bluish ulcers; unconscious. Moaning and **sliding down in the bed** from excessive weakness; lower jaw fallen, **tongue dry, leathery and shrunken to a third of its natural size,** and paralyzed; pulse weak and intermittent. It is hardly possible to draw a picture of a more **desperate case of typhoid than this.**

Dr. E.B. Nash

NATRIUM CARB.: Weakness of the ankles from childhood, finds a good remedy in *Natrum carb.*

Dr. E.B. Nash

NATRIUM MUR.: Mapped tongue is found under *Natrium mur., Arsenicum alb., Lachesis, Nitric acid,* and *Taraxacum.*

Dr. E.B. Nash

NATRIUM MUR.: If the **upper lip** is much thickened or swollen, not of an erysipelatous character, we would think of three remedies, all of which have it, *Belladonna, Calcarea ost., Natrum mur.*

Dr. E.B. Nash

NATRIUM MUR.: It not only removes the tendency to intermittent, but restores the patient to health, and takes away the tendency to colds—**the susceptibility to colds, and to periodicity.** It is the **susceptibility** that is removed. We know that every attack predisposes to another attack. Each attack of ague is more destructive than the previous one. The drugs used increase the susceptibility; the homeopathic remedy removes the susceptibility. **Homeopathic treatment tends to simplify the human economy** and to make disease more easily managed. Unless this susceptibility be eradicated, man goes down lower and lower into emaciation from above downwards.

Dr. J.T. Kent

NATRIUM SULPH.: (Liver) In chronic diarrhea there is almost always some trouble with the liver, evidenced by soreness in right hypochondrium which is **sensitive to touch,** and hurts on walking or any jar.

Dr. E.B. Nash

NATRIUM SULPH: Healthy bile dissolves gall stones in the sac; **healthy urine** does the same to a stone in the pelvis of the kidney.

NITRICUM AC.: The action of this remedy is just as positive upon the **outlet of the alimentary canal.**

Dr. E.B. Nash

OPIUM: Everywhere *Opium* is a producer of insensibility and partial or *complete paralysis* and, other things being equal, is homeopathically indicated there.

Dr. E.B. Nash

PHOSPHORICUM AC.: (Over strain) **It is sin to keep** such young people bowing down to hard study, and while it is true that youth is the time to get an education, it is also true that, it is the time when too **great a strain** in that direction may utterly **wreck** and forever incapacitate a mind which might, with more time and care, have been a blessing to the world.

Dr. E.B. Nash

PSORINUM: So far as prejudice against using such remedies is concerned, **we should be as honest** as was James B. Bell. when he said of psorinum, "whether derived from purest gold or purest filth, our gratitude **for its excellent services** forbids us to enquire or care."

Dr. E.B. Nash

SPONGIA TOST.: (Croup) The cough is dry and sibilant, or sounds like a saw driven through a pine board, each cough corresponding to a **thrust of the saw. Croup** often comes on after **exposure to dry, cold winds.** It generally comes on in the **evening,** with high fever, excitement and fearfulness.

Dr. E.B. Nash

STAPHYSAGRIA: It is one of the best remedies for affections of the **prostate gland in old men,** with frequent urination and dribbling of urine afterwards.

Dr. E.B. Nash

STICTA PUL.: I have found *Sticta* promptly curative in inflammatory **rheumatism of the knee joint.** It is very sudden in its attacks, and unless promptly relieved by *Sticta* it will go on to the exudative stage and become chronic in character.

Dr. E.B. Nash

STICTA PUL.: I have relieved many cases of **chronic catarrh with *Sticta;*** some of years standing.

Dr. E.B. Nash

15. SPECIAL POINTERS
OF SOME REMEDIES

ABSCESS

Calcarea carb. for deep abscesses. These will get absorbed or become calcareous.

Dr. A.N. Mukherji

ACUTE RHEUMATISM

The more **frequent relapses** set in, the more specially is *Mercurius* indicated.

Dr. Boehr

ADENOIDS

I have cured probably 100 cases of *Adenoids* with *Tuberculinum alone.*

Dr. J.T. Kent

AFTER EFFECTS

Pyrogen is sometimes useful when there is a history of septicemia, severe **after effects** of dental **extraction,** or ill-health commencing after an **abortion,** in the absence of any obvious pelvic pathology.

Dr. Foubister

ALMOST SPECIFICS

Homeopathy knows no specifics, except the specific remedy for the individual, yet, as Hahnemann teaches us, some remedies so exactly reproduce a diseased condition, as to become specific. Such are *Cantharis* in cystitis, *Belladonna* in scarlet fever, *Merc. cor. in* dysentery and *Latro. m.,* in angina pectoris.

Dr. M.L. Tyler

ANTIDOTE TO NATRUM

If vertigo and headache be very persistent or prostration be prolonged after *Natrum, Nux vomica* will relieve.

Dr. H.C. Allen

Capsicum is recommended by Hahnemann for home-sickness with flushed cheeks. He has uttered a truth, the correctness of which every practitioner can easily verify if he chooses. (*Ign., Phosphoric acid, Merc. sol.*)

Dr. Jahr

ARTHRITIS

Morgan bacillus is useful in **arthritis,** where nothing else works.

Dr. Robert H. Farley

BALDNESS

Arsenicum is an excellent remedy for **baldness,** if the hair fall out in consequence of an impoverished condition of the follicles, the scalp and the **skin generally are dry,** and the patient's assimilative powers are impaired.

Dr. Charles hempel

ALOPECIA AREATA

I would like to remind you of the efficacy of *Vinca minor* in alopecia areata. Hair fall out and are replaced by grey hair, **bald spot covered with a fine white wooly fuzz.**

Dr. E.A. Farringon

BLEEDING FROM INTESTINES

Ammonium carb. has bleeding from intestines with **each monthly period.**

Dr. Leon Vannier

BLEPHARITIS

Argentum nitricum: In blepharitis, *Graphites* and *Staphysagria* have served me **oftener** than *Argentum nitricum.*

Dr. E.B. Nash

BLISTERS

Blisters on the hands from heavy manual labour **disappear overnight** after the application of 10% *Aristolochia* ointment.

Dr. Julius mezger

BURNS

No home in town or country should be without stinging nettle tincture *Urtica urens* —if only because of its **magic power over** burns; for almost instant relief of pain and rapid healing. This applied, of course, to fairly **superficial burns.**

Dr. M.L. Tyler

CANTHARIS

Cantharis internally in homeopathic potency, is a very old tip for charming away the pains of burns.

Dr. M.L. Tyler

CANCER

Hydrastis: I should be content, led by my own experience, that the *Hydrastis* treatment is the very best known for this disease. It **improves the appetite** and condition of the patient generally. Under its use, the complexion alter, the **state of the blood improves.** It marvelously allays the pain of cancer, in this respect, altogether surpassing opium; morphia or any so-called anodyne. **It retards the growth of cancer.**

Dr. Gutteridge

CANCER PAIN

Magnesia phos. **can relieve** the excruciating pain of cancer.

Dr. Heselton

CANCER-ARSENIC

Judging from our own experience, in the debility of cancer, *Hydrastis* **must yield palm to** *Arsenicum,* for we have repeatedly witnessed the most decided improvement from a course of *Arsenicum.*

Dr. Ruddock

CANCER-LIPS

Arsenicum alb. is of great service in epithelioma (cancer) of the nose and lips.

Dr.J.T. Kent

CATALEPSY

Cannabis indica should be remembered if we ever come across a case of catalepsy. In its power of causing catalepsy, its **only rival** is the chloride of tin.

Dr. Hughes

CHOLELITHIASIS

The remedy to cure the condition permanently is *Cinchona*. (**Continue it for a number of months.**)

Dr. E.A. Ferrington

COLLAPSE

Carbo veg. often, at the brink of death, **a saviour** in those state of collapse, dissolution of blood and paralytic conditions, which seem rapidly to involve the whole organism.

Dr. C.G. Raue

CRAMPS

Patients who come to hospital complaining of severe cramps, **especially in calves,** very often have to get either *Cuprum* or *Calcarea*.

Dr. M.L. Tyler

DOG BITE

I always give *Lyssinum* for every dog bite. I have never had, and I have never seen anything, but the **best of results.** It relieves the pain and they never have any bad effects at all. They always heal up; as a routine proposition. I give *Lyssin*.

Dr. A.H. Grimmer

DYSMENORRHOEA

Single dose of the *Magnesia phos.*, cm **just any time** the patient happened to come up, not necessarily during the painful period, have cured for us quite a number of cases.

Dr. M.L. Tyler

EXERTION

Arsenicum is the remedy for debility resulting from over taxing of the muscular tissues, such as follows prolonged exertion, climbing mountains etc.

Dr. E.A. Farrington

EXHAUSTION

Senna is one of the best remedies in the materia medica for **simple exhaustion** with excessive nitrogenous waste.

Dr. E.A. Farrington

FATIGUE

Remember the use of *Coffea* **for fatigue** arising from long journeys, especially **during hot weather.**

Dr. E.A. Farrington

FEVER - CINA

In **lingering remittent** fevers of children, having symptoms of helminthiasis with or without worms, *Cina* **is specific.**

Dr. Chepmall

FILARIASIS

I became convinced that filariasis should be treated as a psoro-syphilitic disease and that *Mercurius sulphuricus* was the appropriate remedy. I tried the same remedy in cases of the same degrees of chronicity, utilising the several potencies of the remedy up to m.m. potency according to the nature of each case, and have succeeded in curing a very large number of cases. Though, this amounts to routine practice, **I consider this remedy as a specific for this particular disease,** and this may be used safely in all cases. In the more chronic cases, **though the swelling has continued for a long time,** the parts have lost their hardness and become soft, and the patients have become free and **normal as general health.**

Dr. T.S. Iyer

GANGLION

I have myself frequently obtained much reduction in the size of the ganglion situated **at the back of the wrist** by the external application of *Benzoic acid* in an ointment.

Dr. Hughes

GASTRITIS

Arsenicum is suitable in **every form,** the mildest to the most severe.

Dr. Boehr

GOUT

The **more *Benzoic acid* is used** in gout, the more it will be prized.

Dr. C. Hering

HAIR FALL

Aloe 6th dilution is reported to have cured falling of hair.

Dr. Ruddock

HECTIC FEVER

Sulphur is to be considered in deep seated sepsis, especially when associated with hectic fever and rigors.

Dr. D.M. Gibson

HEMICRANIA

Sepia may be regarded as an **excellent remedy** for the paroxysms of hemicrania, which constitutes a source of distress to chlorotic females with lively temperaments.

Dr. Bochr

HIGH BLOOD PRESSURE

Adrenalinum 200 to 10m gives me **great results** in what other doctors pronounce high pressure and its results.

Dr. W.A. Yingling

HYDROPHOBIA

I consider *Stramonium* the **nearest** simillimum we have for hydrophobia.

Dr. George Royal

JAUNDICE

Mercurius is a **specific remedy** in a great number of cases of jaundice.

Dr. Laurie

JAUNDICE IN NEWBORN

I think, in desperate cases of jaundice in the newborn babies, *Thyroidin* will bring back the patient almost from the jaws of death.

Dr. Ghosh

LABOUR-PAINS

No remedy can at all be compared with *Gelsemium* Q, 1 to 5 drops, every 30 minutes, to produce relaxation of rigid, unyielding os-uteri in labour.

Dr. Douglas

LUMBAGO

The specific remedy for **lumbago is not** *Pulsatilla,* as was formerly supposed, but *Rhus tox.* So far, I have cured about every case that I have had to treat, with *Rhus tox.* In three to four days, except perhaps two or three cases where I had to **complete the cure with** *Pulsatilla.*

Dr. Jahr

Ordinary lumbago yields very readily to the internal and external use of *Aconite.*

Dr. Hempel

MEMORY

There are few remedies in the entire materia medica having **impaired memory** as so marked a characteristic. In restoring the memory *Anacardium* cures the patient of all other troubles.

Dr. Guernsey

MIASMS

Thuja occidentalis: Hahnemann recognized three miasms (as he called them) which complicated the treatment of all diseases. They were Psora, Sycosis and Syphilis.

Sulphur was his chief anti-psoric, *Mercury* his anti-syphilitic and *Thuja* his anti-sycotic.

Whatever may be said against his theories along this line, certain it is that these three remedies **do correct certain states** of the system which seem to obstruct the curative action of other seemingly well-indicated remedies.

Dr. E.B. Nash

MIGRAINE

In many psoric cases, the **bowel nosodes** are of great use and I think they are frequently neglected; most cases of migraine, used one of the **bowel nosodes** to be cured permanently **although *Tuberculinum*** plays a great part here.

Dr. Quinton

Cannabis indica is the most useful medicine we possess for diminishing the frequency of the **paroxysms of migraine.**

Dr. Ringer

When you are struck with a *Kali bich.* migraine that does not respond **always remember** *Iris.*

Dr. D.M. Borland

MODALITY

As for *Silicea,* this is **cold blooded** in chronic cases, but if a case of *Silicea* is acute or sub-acute, then it is usually, **warm blooded.**

Dr. Ballokossy

MUSCULAR FATIGUE

Arnica should be administered whenever there is muscular fatigue from whatever cause. Its power to aid the respiration of exhausted muscle is truly wonderful.

Dr. Ruddock

NAIL BITE

Dr. Roger in his little synoptic key, gives **three remedies** for nail biting; *Arsenic, Sanicula* and *Hyoscyamus*. I have found *Sanicula* to be most effective in treating that condition.

Dr. Dixon

I think nail biting was due to some nervous irritation. *Ammonium bromatum* is the remedy in the repertory for nail biting. It is the **only one there** and I think it works.

Dr. Gier

NOCTURNAL HEADACHES

Leutic headaches, especially the **nocturnal**, react well with aurums and above all to *Aurum iodatum*.

Dr. Donnar

NON-DEVELOPMENT OF BREAST

In girls, *Lycopodium* is a remedy for amenorrhoea, with **non-development of breasts** in such girls and makes the course appear.

Dr. Leon Renard

PIGEON CHEST

Phosphorus is the only remedy which never fails to cure **pigeon chest;** it should be given for a long time, day and night, at least three months during which time, the chest will be normal.

Dr. E.B. Nash

PRESCRIBING

In taking your case and hunting through your repertories and materia medicas, **don't make the mistake** of getting a remedy too firmly fixed in your mind, or you court disaster.

Dr. Boger

PRINCIPLE PREVAILS

MERCURIUS SOL.: It must be remembered that *Mercury* is no more a panacea for syphilis than is *Sulphur* for psora or *Thuja* for sycosis, else there would be no truth in similia similibus.

Dr. E.B. Nash

PROSTATE CANCER

Use *Cadmium phosphate* in suspected carcinoma of prostate.

Dr. Wilbur K. Bond

REAL TONIC

The only tonic, in the sense of something to impart strength or tone to the human organism, is nourishing food.

Dr. E.B. Nash

GLANDULAR AFFECTION

Drosera can be used as a pathological remedy for **tubercular glands**

Dr. M.L. Tyler

RESISTANCE

Silicea **appears to cause** a leucocytosis and may increase body resistance to disease in this way.

Dr. Ruddock

RESTRAIN

I find *Phosphorus* especially indicated in young men who are trying to restrain their natural sexual passion and yet there is locally erethism. *Phosphorus* **helps** most wonderfully to control this.

Dr. E.A. Farrington

RHEUMATIC PAINS

If a patient complains of rheumatic pains and with it there is present restlessness and **inability to keep quiet,** consider *Thrombidium* before jumping to the conclusion that it is a *Rhus tox.* case.

Homeo. Recorder, Jan. 31

RHEUMATISM

Rheumatism with constipation is a leading indication for Bach's intestinal nosode "Bach polyvalent 200."

Dr. Edward whitmont

RHEUMATOID ARTHRITIS

Many cases of rheumatoid arthritis in women begin at the menopause. Whenever this is the case and the small joints of hands and feet are involved, *Caulophyllum* should be one of the drugs; also in any non-menopausal cases, where uterus and small joints are affected.

Dr. M.L. Tyler

SEA SICKNESS

If you ever get a case of sea sickness and you are in doubt between *Petroleum* and *Tabacum*, which is the other common drug for sea sickness, you almost always get that **occipital headache** as well as the **sea sickness in Petroleum**, and *Tabacum* people have not.

Borax acts in the majority of cases of **air sickness,** because it is **sudden dip** which upsets most people, and particularly their terror of falling. I have had a number of cases in which I have completely stopped air sickness by 3 or 4 doses of *Borax* before they started flying.

Dr. D. M. Borland

SEQUENCE (ACONITE AND BRYONIA)

There is one point of practical importance according to my own opinion, with regard to *Bryonia*, namely that supposing *Aconite* had not preceded it in the treatment of bronchitis and also in the treatment of acute rheumatism, I have almost invariably found that *Bryonia* does not begin to produce its curative action until a few doses of *Aconite* have been first administered.

Dr. Hale

SICK HEADACHE

The sick headaches of women, are a type of case in which a nosode may be required. Although these headaches may be **relieved** by such remedies as *Iris versicolor*, they are not really cured by them, and have a tendency to recur with increasing severity. Such a condition may be permanently cured by *Tuberculinum* **in high potency**, administered at infrequent intervals in between the acute attacks.

Dr. Nemo

SYNOVITIS

Apis acts on the synovial membranes, giving a perfect picture of synovitis, particularly when it affects the knees.

Dr. E.A. Farrington

SLEEPLESSNESS

In the form of ordinary *Camphor* pilules, I have found it an excellent remedy in simple **sleeplessness**.

Dr. J.H. Clarke

STERILITY

Natrum muriaticum in brandy, a table-spoonful in evenings, is said to produce conception, from intercourse the following night. Several surprising examples of this have been related to me.

Dr. Hering

STYES

Staphysagria is an excellent remedy **for styes** which is normally given when *Pulsatilla* **fails.** In my experience, I have found this remedy effective in all cases of styes whether chronic or otherwise in **lower or upper lids;** recurrent styes.

Dr. R.B. Das

SUBSTITUTE

In homeopathy, medicines can never replace each other nor be as good as another.

Dr. Kent, Dr. Hahnemann, Dr. Piere Schmidt

SUN STROKE

Among the remedies for prevention of sun stroke, *Gelsemium* is the most important.

Dr. C.G. Raue

TOOTHACHE

Coffea will remove the severest pains which drive the patients almost frantic; they cry, tremble, do not know what to do; the pain is indescribable; it is momentarily relieved by holding cold water in mouth.

Dr. C.G. Raue

VEGETABLE SULPHUR

Lycopodium can also be an **intermediary remedy** in cases where the correctly selected remedies are no longer effective. Therefore *Lycopodium* is called the vegetable *Sulphur.*

Dr. Med. H. Zulla

WORMS

I have repeatedly killed tape worm with Cina as well as the lumbricoides and ascarides.

Dr. Bayes

REMEDIES

ACONITUM NAP.: There is no better picture in a few words of the *Aconite* fever than is given by **Hering,** "heat, with thirst; hard, full and frequent pulse, anxious, impatience, inappeasable, beside himself, **tossing about with agony.**"

Dr. E.B. Nash

ACONITE: In true carditis, **pericarditis,** *Aconite* 30 in watery solution; generally accomplishes everything that can be desired.

Dr. Jahr

ADRENALINUM: *Adrenaline* 200 gave dramatic relief in acute **bronchial asthma** and 1m also palliates, but *Arsenicum alb.*, **to be followed for weakness.**

Homeo. Recorder Feb., 24

ALUMINA: It is one of the best remedies for haemorrhages of the bowels in **typhoid fever.**

Dr. E.B. Nash

ANACARDIUM ORI.: If you find a mydriasis on the left side, this should make you look for *Anacardium.*

Dr. Med. Milar Deichmann

ANTIMONIUM CRUD.: Arthritis deformans responds to *Antimonium crud.* and it is a near specific.

Dr. Schwarts

ANTIMONIUM CRUD.: "Copious haemorrhage from the bowels, mixed with solid faeces; chronic redness of the eyelids; toothache in decayed teeth, worse at night; gastric trouble **after acids,** sour wine, vinegar," etc.

Dr. E.B. Nash

ANTIMONIUM CRUD.: In the form of diarrhea, oftenest with old people, which **alternates** with constipation, *Antimonium crudum* is the only remedy.

Dr. M.L. Tyler

ANTIMONIUM CRUD.: (Digestion) It is especially to be considered if the **gastric derangement is of recent date.** The process of digestion is hardly under way; the eructations taste of the food as he ate it, and the sufferer feels as if he must "throw up" before there will be any relief. In such a case, a few pellets of *Antimonium crudum* on the tongue will **often settle the business, save the loss of a meal,** and all further suffering.

Dr. E.B. Nash

ANTIMONIUM TART.: (Nausea) The nausea of this remedy is as intense as that of *Ipecacuanha*, but not so persistent, and there is **relief after vomiting.** I have found it nearest a specific (of course, we know, there is no absolute specific for any disease) for **cholera morbus** of any remedy. For more than 25 years, I have seldom found it necessary to use any other, and then, only when there were severe **cramps in the stomach** and bowels, when *Cuprum metallicum* relieved.

Dr. E.B. Nash

ANTIMONIUM TART.: (Coarse rattling) If *Antimonium tart.* possessed only the one power of curing that it does, upon the respiratory organs, it would be indispensable. No matter what the name of the trouble, **whether it be bronchitis,** pneumonia, whooping cough or asthma, if there is great accumulation of mucus with **coarse rattling,** of filling up with it, but, at the same time, there seems to be inability to raise it, tartar emetic is the first remedy to be thought of. This is true in all ages and constitutions, but particularly so in children and old people.

Dr. E.B. Nash

ARGENTUM NIT.: Also in epilepsy or convulsions; in the former, (epilepsy) one characteristic symptom is **that, for hours or days before the attack, the pupils are dilated;** in the latter, the convulsions are preceded for a short time by **great restlessness.**

Dr. E.B. Nash

ARGENTUM NIT.: (Back pain) "Pain in the back (small of) relieved when standing or walking, but severe when rising from a seat," is a condition often found in practice. I have often relieved it with *Sulphur* or *Causticum,* but **remember also** *Argentum nitricum.*

Dr. E. B. Nash

ARGENTUM NIT.: (Child looks old) Guernsey says, "we think of this remedy on seeing a **withered and dried up person,** made so by disease." This especially in children. "He looks like a little withered old man." (*Fluoric acid,* young people look old) *Argentums* **like gold,** profoundly affects the mind.

Dr. E.B. Nash

ARGENTUM NIT.: It cures **claustro-phobia.**

Dr. M.L. Tyler

ARNICA: (Restores sleep) Sleeplessness caused by over-exertion and extreme weariness of mind or body. Here *Arnica* never fails to summon for the tired, Nature's sweet restorer of balmy sleep.

Dr. M.L. Tyler

ARNICA MONT.: The strong tincture of *Arnica*, applied to **wasp sting,** relieves the pain, and swelling, and in a couple of hours, the sting is forgotten.

Dr. M.L. Tyler

ARSENICUM ALB.: In every one of these affections, ranging along the whole length of the anal, and from the lightest grade of irritation to the most intense inflammatory and **malignant** forms of disease, we will be apt to find everywhere present the **characteristic burning** of this remedy, in greater or lesser degree; and the not less characteristic **amelioration** from heat, and also, though not quite so invariably, the **midnight aggravation.**

Dr. E.B. Nash

ARSENICUM ALB.: Patient is **weak out of proportion** to the rest of his trouble.

Dr. E.B. Nash

ARSENICUM ALB.: (Wrong prescribing) **I do not think** this is sound reasoning or good advice, for **I have never found any rule** by which I could decide from the beginning that a case would later on develop into a case of the **pernicious or malignant** character, which ever call for the exhibition of *Arsenic*.

Dr. E. B. Nash

ARSENICUM ALB.: In **cancrum oris** and severe forms of **aphthae** and generally in malignant **inflammations** and phagedenic conditions of the parts, *Arsenicum* has no rival.

Dr. Hering

BACILLINUM: An inter-current course of Bacillinum will often make wonderful change in patient who has a personal or family history of **chest affections.**

Dr. J.H. Clarke

BACCILLUS MORG: It has removed superficial congestive **swellings of the hands and feet** where no definite pathology would account for it.

Dr. William B. Griggs

BELLADONNA (Throat): **No remedy has greater affinity for the throat.** The burning, dryness (*Sabadilla*), sense of constriction (constant desire to swallow to relieve the sense of dryness, *Lyssinum*), with or without swelling of the palate and tonsils, is sometimes intense. I once witnessed a case of poisoning in which these symptoms were terribly distressing.

Dr. E.B. Nash

BELLIS PER.: In the giddiness of elderly people (cerebral stasis), *Bellis per.,* acts well and does permanent good.

Dr. Burnett

BERBERIS VUL.: No matter what ails the patient, if he has persistent pain in the **region of the kidneys,** do not forget *Berberis vulgaris.*

Dr. E.B. Nash

BERBERIS VUL.: (Arthritis) It is especially to be thought of in arthritic and **rheumatic affections,** when these back symptoms, **connected with urinary alterations are present.** One very characteristic symptom is a burning sensation in the region of the kidneys. Another is **soreness** in region of kidneys when jumping out of a wagon or stepping hard downstairs or from any jarring movement.

Dr. E.B. Nash

BISMUTHUM (Vomit): The body surface is warm and often covered with **warm sweat.** The face is deathly pale, with **rings around** the eyes. This is a perfect picture of *Bismuth,* and no other remedy need be confounded with it.

Dr. E.B. Nash

BRYONIA ALB. (Dryness): With *Bryonia,* it is **excessive dryness or lack of secretion in them.** It begins in the lips, which are parched, dry and cracked, and only ends with the rectum and stools, which are hard and dry as if burnt.

Dr. E.B. Nash

BRYONIA ALB.: It makes no difference what the name of the disease, if the patient feels greatly, ameliorated by lying still and suffers greatly on the **slightest motion,** and the more and **longer he moves the more he suffers,** *Bryonia* is the first remedy to be thought of, and there must be very strong counter-indications along other lines that will rule it out.

Dr. E.B. Nash

BRYONIA ALB. (Stitching pains): The characteristic pains of inflammatory affections of the serous membranes are stitching pains; this is the reason why *Bryonia* comes to be such a real remedy in **pleuritis, meningitis, peritonitis,**

pericarditis, etc. The subjective symptoms corresponding to the remedy must go down before it, and the objectives must as surely follow.

Dr. E.B. Nash

BURSITIS: *Sticta pulmonaria* has been found to be of great efficacy.

Dr. E.C. Price

CALCAREA OSTREARUM: Sensations of **coldness in single parts** should always call to mind *Calcarea ost.,* as well as general coldness. (*Cisus* and *Heloderma.*)

Dr. E.B. Nash

CALCAREA PHOS.: The phosphorus element in this preparation seems to change the temperament, for while it retains its wonderful remedial power over **tardy bone development, it acts best in spare (lean) subjects** instead of fat. So that if we find a sickly child with fontanelles remaining open too long or re-opening after once closed, the child being spare and anaemic, we think of this remedy.

Dr. E.B. Nash

CALADIUM SEG.: According to the experience of others and my own Caladium is the most efficient remedy in **pruritus vulvae.**

Dr. C.G. Raue

CANTHARIS: *Cantharis* will relieve the raw burning pain and promotes healing; covers **acute nephritis** which may ensue.

Dr. Charles C. Boericke

CARBO AN.: The subjects of it are often disposed to **glandular swellings,** indurations and suppurations.

Dr. E.B. Nash

CARBO VEG.: Coldness of the knees, even in bed (*Apis*); of left arm and left leg; very cold hands and feet; **fingernails blue.**

Dr. E.B. Nash

CAUSTICUM: *Causticum* also has very marked action upon the urinary organs, as is shown by the following symptoms; **"Itching of the orifice of the urethra."** "Constant ineffectual desire to urinate, frequent evacuations of only a few drops, with spasms in the rectum and constipation."

This is like *Nux vomica* and *Cantharis*, and I once cured a **chronic case of cystitis** in a married woman, which had baffled the best efforts of several old school physicians, eminent for their skill, for years.

Dr. E.B. Nash

CAUSTICUM: "He **urinates so easily** that he is not sensible of the stream, and **scarcely believes in the dark that he is urinating at all,** until he makes sure by sense of touch."

Dr. E.B. Nash

CAUSTICUM (Flu and cough): In influenza or what is now called La Grippe, it disputes for first place with *Eupatorium perf.* and *Rhus tox.* All three have a tired, sore, bruised sensation all over the body, and all have soreness in the chest when **coughing,** but if **involuntary micturition is present** *Causticum* wins.

Dr. E.B. Nash

CAUSTICUM: No homeopath can afford to be without an understanding of *Causticum* upon the **respiratory organs.**

Dr. E.B. Nash

CHAMOMILLA: In the chamomilla case, the patient is **exceedingly sensitive to the pain** and exclaims continually, **"Oh, I cannot bear the pain."** Many times have I met this condition in labor cases, and in the majority of them the cross, peevish, snappish, condition of mind accompanying, and seen it changed in a short time to a mild, uncomplaining, patient state, by a single dose of *Chamomilla* 200th.

Dr. E.B. Nash

CHAMOMILLA: It was in my earlier practice, when I was prescribing for names more than I do now, and of course he got *Aconite, Bryonia* and *Rhus toxicodendron*, etc., but no relief. A wiser man was called in consultation and the patient was quickly cured by *Chamomilla.* When I asked the counsel what led him to prescribe this remedy, he answered, **numbness with the pains.**

Dr. E.B. Nash

CHELIDONIUM MAJ.: If we should find pressive pain in the region of the liver, whether it be, enlarged and sensitive to pressure or not, bitter taste in the mouth, tongue coated thickly yellow, with red margins showing imprint of the teeth, **yellowness of whites of eyes,** face, hands and skin; stools gray, clay coloured, or yellow as gold, **urine also yellow** as gold, lemon coloured or dark brown, leaving a yellow colour on vessel when emptied out, **loss of appetite,** disgust and nausea, or vomiting of bilious matter, and especially if patient could retain nothing but **hot drinks on the stomach,** we would have a clear case for *Chelidonium,* even though the infra-scapular pain were absent. All these symptoms might be found in either a chronic or acute case.

Dr. E.B. Nash

CLEMATIS EREC.: Dreamy state, indifference to disease, and even death; **absence of efforts to get well,** absence of interest in the present, utter complacency to future and drowsy state indicates Clematis arecto flora.

Dr. Hughes

COFFEA CRUD.: Hering used to recommend *Aconite* and *Coffea* in **alternation in painful inflammatory affection,** where the fever symptoms of the former and also the nervous sensibility of the latter were present, and I know, of no two remedies that alternate better, **though I never do it, since I learned to closely individualize.**

Dr. E.B. Nash

CUPRUM MET.: Dunham said, "in *Camphor*, **collapse** is most prominent; in *Veratrum album*, the **evacuation** and vomiting; in *Cuprum*, **the cramps."**

Dr. E.B. Nash

DROSERA (Glands): In *Drosera* gland cases, one notices not only the diminution in the size of the gland, but that the **old scars fade away,** get free and come to the surface, that discolouration goes, and that when a gland does break down under *Drosera*, it behaves in a very restrained manner, with a small opening. Little discharge and that it leaves practically nothing to mark what has taken place.

Dr. M.L. Tyler

DROSERA ROT.: I found that the prolonged use of *Drosera* induces tuberculization in animals and its power to cure tuberculization never fails me.

Dr. Curie

EUPHRASIA: (Face) *Euphrasia* has a shining face which looks as if it had been varnished, the skin of the face **cracks as varnish does.** The face feels stiff.

Dr. H.A. Roberts

FERRUM MET.: It is true that **when iron is introduced** into the system in large quantities with a view to supplying a deficiency of iron in the blood **that it is not assimilated,** but may be almost entirely obtained from the faeces, having been eliminated by the intestines.

Dr. E.B. Nash

GELSEMIUM SEMP. (headache): One notable characteristic is that, sometimes the **headache is relieved by a profuse flow** of urine. (*Lac defloratum* has a profuse flow of urine during sick headache to which it is adapted, **but the pain is not so markedly relieved by the flow.**)

Dr. E.B. Nash

HEPAR SULPH.: (Asthma) The *Hepar* asthma is worse in dry cold air and **better in damp,** while *Natrum sulph.* is exactly the **opposite like *Dulcamara*.** There is no other remedy that I know that has the **amelioration so strongly in damp weather** as *Hepar sulphur.*

Dr. E.B. Nash

HYDRASTIS CAN.: Dr. Logan reported the successful treatment of more than 200 cases of diphtheria with *Hydrastis* gargle.

Dr. Ruddock

IPECACUANHA: The spasmodic cough and asthma do not seem to all depend upon accumulation of mucus, for *Ipecacuanha* is often our best remedy in the **first stage of both** asthma and whooping cough, **before the stage, when the mucus is present.**

Dr. E.B. Nash

Nash-about himself: In what I have written, **I do not pretend to have told,** all, and if I thought that any young physician would be led to rely alone upon this work of mine or be led away from thorough study of the material medica, instead of to it, I would stop writing.

Dr. E.B. Nash

ALTERNATIVE: A medicine which gradually induces a **change in the habit or constitution,** and restores healthy functions without sensible evacuation.

Dr. E.B. Nash

KALIUM MUR.: Is a well proven **anti-infective and anti-virus** remedy.

Dr. Koppikar

LAC CAN.: If the **breasts and throat** get sore during menstruation, especially if the **menses flow in gushes** instead of continuously, *Lac caninum* is the remedy.

Dr. E.B. Nash

LACHESIS: Its action is perfectly homeopathic to acute **yellow atrophy of the liver.**

Dr. Jausset

LACHESIS: Exceptional loquacity, with rapid change of subjects; jumps abruptly from one idea to another.

Dr. E.B. Nash

LACHESIS: Hempel wrote in his first volume of materia medica: "in spite of every effort to the contrary, the conviction has gradually forced itself upon my mind that the pretended pathogenesis of *Lachesis,* which has emanated from Dr. Hering's otherwise meritorious and highly praise worthy efforts, **is a great delusion,** and that with the exception of the poisonous effects with which this publication is abundantly mingled the balance of the symptoms, are unreliable."

Hempel **modified his views somewhat,** I think, in later editions.

Dr. E.B. Nash

LILIUM TIG.: The **uterine symptoms are sometimes** marked so as to be over-looked for the time by the **violence of the heart symptoms.**

Dr. E.B. Nash

LYCOPODIUM: Loose Velt said that, a **half open condition of the eyes** during sleep pointed to *Lycopodium.*

Dr. Sidwick

LYCOPODIUM: It is particularly adopted to the treatment of **cirrhosis of the liver.**

Dr. Boehr

LYCOPODIUM: It has often saved neglected, mal-treated or imperfectly **cured cases of pneumonia from running into consumption.**

Dr. E.B. Nash

LYCOPODIUM: If you find corresponding failure in the sensorium of **old men,** the **memory fails,** they use wrong words to express themselves, mix things up, generally in writing, spelling, and are, in short, unable to do ordinary mental work on account of failing brain power, remember *Lycopodium.*

Dr. E.B. Nash

LYCOPODIUM: A feeling of **satiety** is found under this remedy which alternates with a feeling of **hunger** of a peculiar kind.

Dr. E.B. Nash

LYCOPODIUM: The liver troubles of *Lycopodium* are more apt to be of the **atrophic variety,** while those of *China* are **hypertrophic,** both being equally useful in their sphere.

Lycopodium has almost, if not quite, as marked action upon the **urinary organs as upon the liver.**

Dr. E.B. Nash

MERCURIUS: No remedy has this **condition of mouth** in any degree equal to *Mercury.*

Dr. E.B. Nash

MERCURIUS COR.: (Eyes) It seems, according to the testimony of others, to be a useful remedy for catarrhal affections of the eyes and nose. Here also, I have no testimony to offer, but would not cast doubt upon it for that reason. **I do not desire to place my own experience ahead of that of others. We are co-laborers. Let each add to the general store of medical knowledge,** that all may draw freely from it as occasion demands.

Dr. E.B. Nash

MERCURIUS COR.: For elongated uvula causing trouble, apply a little of low trituration of *Mercurius corrosivus* on uvula, and it will relieve immediately and permanently.

Dr. R.B. Das

MERCURIUS SOL.: The glands and bones also come strongly under the influence of this remedy. **The glandular swellings** are cold, inclined to suppurate, having these **chilly creepings** afore mentioned. These with the **bone-pains** in the exostoses and caries are all **aggravated at night,** in the warmth of the bed.

Dr. E.B. Nash

MURIATICUM AC.: Cures the muscular weakness following excessive use of opium and tobacco. (*Veratrum alb., Pulsatilla, Avena sativa, Ipecac.*)

Dr. H.C. Allen

NATRIUM CARB.: (Lack of reaction) It was sometimes very effective in cases which displayed very **little reaction,** especially in elderly people.

Dr. Alva Benjamin

NATRIUM MUR.: (Anaemia) I have seen better cures of bad cases of anemia by *Natrum muriaticum* in potentized form, than I ever did from iron in any form, although iron has its cases, as have also *Pulsatilla, Cyclamen, Calcarea phos., Carbo veg., China* and many other remedies.

Dr. E.B. Nash

NATRIUM MUR.: *Natrum mur.* also cures the headaches of school girls, and here it may be difficult to choose between it and *Calcarea phos.*, both remedies also being particularly adapted to **anaemic states.** Indeed, I have sometimes missed and had to give *Calcarea phos.* When *Natrium* failed and vice versa, because I could not make the choice.

Dr. E.B. Nash

NATRIUM MUR.: (Diabetes) Of course, the intense thirst of salt is well known, and keeps pace with the **hunger.** Now, this is the **case with diabetes,** for which *Natrum* is a curative if otherwise indicated. In all of these cases, of course, it must **be used high,** for we get the low in our food.

Dr. E.B. Nash

NATRIUM SULPH.: (Root of nails) One point in the digestive upset of *Natrium sulph.* is that whether it is a gall bladder or liver upset or whether it is an appendix, concurrently with the attack, the patients are liable to get a **suppurative condition about the root of the nails.** I have verified it several times. A patient with chronic liver trouble, who, whenever he is getting a slight increase of disturbance, begins to develop suppurating places round his nails, will very often run to *Natrum sulphuricum.*

Dr. D.M. Borland

NUX VOMICA (Stomach): The pressure **as from a stone, occurs also** under *Bryonia* and *Pulsatilla.*

Dr. E.B. Nash

OPIUM: I will say just here that, any homeopathic physician that feels obliged to use *Opium* or its alkaloid in this way and for this purpose, does not understand his business and had better study his materia medica, and the principles of applying it according to Hahnemann, or else go over to the **old school where they make no pretensions to have any law of cure.** In the first place, *Opium* in narcotic doses **does not produce sleep, but stupor,** and it only relieves pain by rendering the patient unconscious to it. How many cases have been so **masked by such treatment,** that the disease progressed until there was no chance of cure? **Pain, fever and all other symptoms are the voice of the disease, telling where is the trouble and guiding us to the remedy.**

Dr. E.B. Nash

PHOSPHORICUM AC. (weakness): Let us remember that the profound **weakness and depression** of *Phosphoric acid,* is upon the **sensorium and nervous system,** and will be there whether diarrhea is present or not. It is markedly so in typhoids, so I can fully attest from abundant observation.

Dr. E.B. Nash

PHYTOLACCA DEC.: (milk) When a mother says, she has **no milk or that the milk is scanty,** thicker, unhealthy, dries up soon, *Phytolacca* becomes then a constitutional remedy if there are no contra indicating symptoms.

Dr. J.T. Kent

PICRICUM ACID: In any psychoneurotic group of patients, there are those with present fatigue, **worse in the morning,** who say they feel more tired on arising than they went to bed, and also mention that the **least desk** work leaves them dragged out and listless, I will now give more thought to *Picric acid.*

Dr. Robert L. Redfield

PLUMBUM MET.: (Jaundice) H. Guernsey claimed great powers for it in jaundice; whites of eyes, skin, stool and urine, all are **very yellow,** and I have prescribed it with success.

Dr. E.B. Nash

PSORINUM: (Modality) I have found at least several times that a remedy like *Psorinum* which is so terribly chilly, is necessary in the course of treatment of deep allergies, inspite of the fact that the patient is very warm blooded.

Dr. Schmidt

PSORINUM (Three miasms): I have cured eruptions on the skin resembling itch with *Psorinum*, rheumatic troubles that were very obstinate under our usual remedies with *Medorrhinum* and a long standing case of caries of the spine with *Syphilinum*, but **in not one of these cases had the patient, that I could trace, itch, gonorrhoea or syphilis.**

Dr. E.B. Nash

PULSATILLA - CYCLAMEN: If a case seems to be *Pulsatilla*, but the mental state is peevish and irritable, rather than mild, try *Cyclamen*. It will often work wonders.

Homeo. Recorder, Aug.31

PULSATILLA: The bad taste in the mouth is persistent and the loss of taste is frequent, as is also the **loss of smell.**

Dr. E.B. Nash

PULSATILLA: The hemorrhages flow, and stop, and flow again; **continually changing.** The stools in diarrhea constantly change in colour; they are green, yellow, white, watery or slimy; as Guernsey expresses it, **"no two stools alike."**

Dr. E.B. Nash

RADIUM BROM.: All carcinomas I have to treat now, who have had x-rays, I put on to one of the radio active salts as a first measure to try to **antidote the x-rays.** Usually I use one of the radium salts, either radium bromide or radium iodide. If I can find any indication for iodine, I prefer the radium iodide, to radium bromide.

Dr. E.M. Borland

RHUS TOX.: For instance, in *Rhus tox.*, the **loose cough is worse in the morning,** tight, **dry one in the evening.**

Dr. E.B. Nash

RHUS TOX. (Urticaria): Great **Sensitiveness to open air;** putting the hand from under the bedcover brings on the cough (*Bar., Hepar.*)

Pain between the shoulders on swallowing.

Cough during chill; dry, teasing, fatiguing, **but urticaria over body during heat.**

Dr. E.B. Nash

RHUS TOX. (Lumbago): Indeed *Rhus tox.* is one of our best remedies in lumbago.

Dr. E.B. Nash

RHUS TOX.: (fevers): Whenever in fevers or even inflammatory diseases, the sensorium becomes cloudy (smoky) or stupefaction sets in, with low grade of muttering delirium, dry tongue, etc., we think of *Rhus tox.*

Dr. E.B. Nash

SABAL SERR.: Saw palmetto, besides its well written up action on the **prostate gland,** can now take its stand as a beautifying remedy, since it promotes in a marked degree, the growth of the **mammary gland in women.**

Dr. Dewey

SACCHARUM LACTIS: It is a remedy introduced by Dr. Swan. It was his **'Fatigue powder,'** the accuracy of which I have verified.

Dr. Ying ling

SANGUINARIA CAN.: Sometimes indicated after *Sulphur* and *Lachesis* have failed, especially if the circumscribed **redness of the cheeks appears.**

Dr. E.B. Nash

SANGUINARIA CAN.: It is decidedly homeopathic in **acute gastritis.**

Dr. Dewey

SARSAPARILLA: In *Sarsaparilla,* the **neck emaciates** and skin (in general) **lies in folds.**

Dr. E.B. Nash

SEPIA: The best remedy we have for **small ulcers** about the points of **fingers is Sepia.**

Dr. E. A. Farrington

SEPIA: A history of **bed wetting in early life** is a good pointer to *Sepia*.

Dr. T. Douglas Ross

SEPIA (Toothache): It is essential to ascertain the **seat of the local disease** with accuracy; for; every experienced homeopath knows how in toothache for instance, it is necessary to select the remedy which in its provings has repeatedly **acted upon the very tooth that suffers.** The specific curative power of *Sepia* in those stubborn and sometimes fatal joint abscesses of the fingers and toes, is extraordinary conclusive evidence upon this point, for they **differ from similar gathering in location only,** while the remedies so suitable **for abscess elsewhere remain ineffectual here.**

Dr. Boger

SEPIA: A short walk fatigues her very much. She faints easily from extremes of cold or heat, after getting wet, from riding in a carriage, while kneeling at church, and on other trifling occasion.

Dr. E.B. Nash

SILICEA: It is chiefly when scrofula manifests itself in the **bones and joints** that *Silicea* proves its powers.

Dr. Hughes

SILICEA: The first great property of *Silicea* is its power over **suppuration.**

Dr. Hughes

SILICEA: Promotes expulsion of foreign bodies from the tissues, fish bones, needles, bone splinters.

Dr. E.B. Nash

SPIGELIA ANTII.: I treated in gumpendorf hospital at Vienna, 57 cases of **rheumatic carditis** with one death and *Spigelia* was the only medicine employed.

Dr. Flaishman

SULPHUR: Experience has shown that a vitaminitic troubles, arising from eating **too much cooked meat** are best treated with *Sulphur.*

Dr. F.H. Bellokossy

SULPHUR: I now come to an attempt to give some idea of the curative sphere of Hahnemann's **king of anti-psorics.** I do not, in this place feel it incumbent upon me to enter into a defence of Hahnemann's psora theory against those who discard it **because they do not understand and profit by it.** There is no need of such defence. The truth stands confirmed (with those who have put to the test Hahnemann's rules for the use of *Sulphur*) that, it has **power to overcome certain obstacles to the usual action of drugs** when indicated by the symptoms, or least seemingly so. That is the reason why the indication as laid down in the books reads; **"when seemingly indicated drugs do not cure, use *Sulphur*,"** because psora is the obstacle to be overcome.

Dr. E.B. Nash

SULPHUR: Let no one understand that *Sulphur* is the only remedy capable of removing psoric complications, but simply that *Sulphur* will be likely to be oftened here, because it oftener covers the usual manifestations of **psora in its pathogenesis** than any other remedy. There are anti psorics, like *Psorinum, Causticum, Graphites,* etc., which may have to be used instead of *Sulphur.* And we know which one by the same law which guides us in selection of the right remedy any time.

Dr. E.B. Nash

SULPHUR (Absorption): There is one thing about Sulphur that is often underestimated by the profession in general, viz., **its power of absorption.** It is after the state of effusion has set in or even later when this stage is passed and the results of the inflammatory process are to be gotten rid of; like, the **enlargement of the joints in rheumatism,** exudations into serous sacs, pleura, meningeal membranes, peritoneum, etc. *Bryonia* is one of the remedies first thought of in these cases, and we have another remedy that is making a record for itself here, viz., *Kali muriaticum*, but, when the case is complicated by psora and especially, when the characteristic **burnings** stand out prominently *Sulphur* is **almost sure to be needed before the case is finished**.

Dr. E.B. Nash

SULPHUR (Circulation): *Sulphur* seems to have the power of **equalizing the circulation** in persons subject to such local congestions and inflammations.

Dr. E.B. Nash

SULPHUR: Every time she urinates, she jumps from a sharp pain, as if a sharp instrument had been stuck under the **great toe nail.**

Dr. H.A. Roberts

SULPHUR (knee): We may use *Sulphur* in synovitis, particularly after exudation has taken place. *Sulphur* here produces absorption and very rapidly too, particularly **in the knee.**

Dr. E.A. Farrington

SYPIIILINUM: I have wasted much time trying to find a remedy in cases with tuberculosis in the family. Now, I like very much, to augment *Tuberculinum* with *Syphilinum*.

Dr. Wilbur K. Bond

THERIDION CUR. (Caries): In rachitis, caries and necrosis, *Theridion curassavicum* apparently goes to the root of the evil and destroys the cause.

Dr. Baruch

THERIDION CUR.: Give *Theridion curassavicum* for the vertigo and nausea associated with **abscess of the liver.**

Dr. Lippe

TROMBIDIUM MUS. (Nose drip): There are many people whose noses will begin to drip, the minute they begin to eat, a fluent discharge from the nose. It is exceedingly annoying to the patient. I have at several occasions, been able to relieve that entirely by *Trombidium*.

Dr. H.A. Roberts

TUBERCULINUM BOV.: A person running down, never finding the right remedy, or relief only momentarily, has a constant desire to change, to travel, to go somewhere and **do something different.** That **cosmopolitan** condition of mind belongs strongly to the one who needs *Tuberculinum*.

Dr. Burnett.

URTICA UREMS: It has cured **obstinate cases of deltoid rheumatism** in 10 drop doses of the tincture. It is thought that this has the power to dissolve deposits of urates in the muscules.

Dr. Dewey

VANADIUM MET.: Burnett termed *Vanadium* his 'sheet anchor' in fatty **changes of the liver;** also declares, it meets the antheroma of the brain or liver to a nicety; real remedy of this organic change, and mentions *Bellis perennis* as a complementary remedy. From slight experience with the remedy, this I can well believe. He claims that these two remedies have restored veritable physical wrecks to health.

Dr. Donnar

VIPERA BER.: It is the valuable remedy in brachia neuritis where it was noted that the patient **supported the arm of the affected side to get relief.**

Dr. Robert L. Redfield

WIESBADEN (Hairfall): By use of this remedy, the hair will grow rapidly and become darker in cases of falling of hair. Give in 200 dilution.

Dr. R.B. Das

16. SOME WIDER UNIVERSAL PRINCIPLES AND THE (CAUSE OF) UNCERTAIN RESULTS IN HOMEOPATHY

(ALSO RELATIVE IMPORTANCE OF SYMPTOMS, MODALITIES AND CLINICAL EXPERIENCES)

AFFECTIONS AND INTELLIGENCE

Think what a state it is for a man who has been in good condition of health, respected in his business circles, to have a desire to commit suicide. The man's intellectual nature keeps the man in contact with the world; but his **affections are largely kept to himself.** A man can have affection for all sorts of things and perversion of the affections, but his intellect will guide him not to show his likes and dislikes to the world. The affections can not be seen, **but man's intellect is subject to inspection.** He cannot conceal his intellect.

Dr. J.T. Kent

The mental symptoms can be classified in a remedy. The things that relate to the memory are not so important as also the **things that relate to the intelligence are not so important as the things that relate to the affections or desire and aversions.**

Dr. J.T. Kent

ALTERNATING STATUS

We sometimes do not discover this alternation of states until we have brought it back two or three times by incorrect prescribing.

Dr. J.T. Kent

ANXIETY AND SLEEPLESSNESS

In sleeplessness from anxiety, restlessness, anguish, fear; when man, woman or child tosses feverishly in despair of ever getting off to sleep, *Aconite* **is simply scientific magic.**

Dr. M.L. Tyler

ARTHRITIS

Remember *Causticum* in those difficult rheumatoid cases of arthritis, where there are deformities and contractions, and the patient **suffers more in cold, dry winds and less in warm wet days.**

Dr. M.L. Tyler

BLAME ON HOMEOPATHY

Homeopathy is too often blamed, when the blame lies in the **stupidity of the prescriber.**

Dr. E.B. Nash

BOILS

Tarentula or *Anthracinum* clear up the boils in a few days brilliantly and miraculously. (*Hepar, Bell., Arn., Silicea*).

Dr. Dorothy Shephered

CANCER

Any case of cancer complicated by a weak heart or diseased kidneys can hardly get well, because the reaction to curative remedy will kill such a patient in a comparatively short time.

Dr. A.H. Grimmer

Do not dwell upon the cancer, for it is not the cancer but the patient that you are treating. It is the patient that is sick, and whenever a patient is sick enough to have a cancer, his state of order is too much disturbed to be cured.

Dr. J.T. Kent

CAUSE OF ALARM

If inward affections work outward towards the surface, there is not usually cause for alarm, but if they go the other way, look out for breakers, there is shipwreck ahead.

Dr. E.B. Nash

CLINICAL TESTIMONY

You do not get all these things in the text, you have to see them applied, but the things that I give you, that are brought out clinically, are those things that have come from applying the symptoms of the remedy at the bed side of the sick folks.

Dr. J.T. Kent

CONSCIENCE OF PHYSICIAN

It is quite a profitable business for one who has not much conscience and not much intelligence. But a conscientious physician feels worried and knows he is not doing what he ought to do to his patient, unless he reaches out for the remedy which **touches the constitution.**

Dr. J.T. Kent

CONSTITUTIONAL STATE

If the patient has a good constitutional state, he will get over the cold by the **acute remedy, but the old gouty,** rheumatic, flabby patients **need a constitutional remedy.**

Dr. J. T. Kent

COUGH

Ammonium carb. has **cured the cough of influenza when** everything else has failed, and I have more than once not found it **necessary to give a second dose.**

Dr. Younam

CRISIS AT THREE STAGES

Teething is a crisis and the things that are within will come out all the time, just as there are troubles that are likely to come out at the time of **puberty** and at the **climacteric** period.

Dr. J.T. Kent

CURE

You can only cure the patients if they desire to reform, and if you can inspire them to live a better life. Without this you cannot save them, and those who take delight in such things are not worth saving, and medicine will not take hold of them. To cure, the patient must use his will to help the remedy.

Dr. J. T. Kent

DANGER-SYCOTIC PATIENT

The psoric patient has many uncomfortable sensations, such as sharp cutting, neuralgic pains about the heart; those patients think they are about to die and want to lie down and keep quiet, but there is no danger; **it is the sycotic and syphilitic heart patients who die suddenly without warning.**

Dr. H.A. Roberts

DESIRES AND IMPULSES

An impulse is sometimes overwhelming and over balances the mind, and he commits suicide. Some persons lie awake at night and long for death, and there is no reason for it. That is the state of the will, insanity of the will. **Desires are of the will; impulses come into the thoughts.** If he desires to have a knife to commit suicide, that is altogether different from an impulse to commit suicide.

Dr. J. T. Kent

DIAGNOSIS AND REMEDY

Failure to diagnose may wreck the physician **while diagnosis without the remedy** is poor consolation for the patient.

Dr. M.L. Tyler

DISCHARGES-A REALITY

The woman feels best when she has more or less of **leucorrhoeas as it seems a sort of protection.** These discharges that we meet every day are dried up and controlled by local treatments, by washes, and by local applications of every kind and the patient put into the hands of the undertaker, or made a **miserable wreck.** If these catarrhal patients are not healed from within outwards, the discharges had better be allowed to go on. While these discharges exist, the patient is comfortable.

Dr. J. T. Kent

EYEBROW

When *Kali carb.* fails, *Anatherum* may be tried in falling of hair from eyebrows.

Dr. R.B. Das

FACE — THE INDEX OF MIND

The study of the faces of people is very profitable. It is profitable to study the faces of wealthy people so that you may be able to judge their intentions from their facial expressions. A man shows his business of life in his face; he shows his method of thinking, his hatreds, his longings, and his loves. How easy it is to pick out a man who has never loved to do anything but to eat-the **Epicurean face.** How easy it is to pick out a man who has never loved anything but money-the **miserly face.** You can see the love in many of the **professional faces;** you can single out the student's face. These are only manifestations of the love of the life which they live. Some manifest hatred; hatred of the life in which they have been forced to live; hatred of mankind;

hatred of life. in those who have been disappointed to everything they have undertaken to do we see hatred stamped upon the face. We see these things in remedies just as we see them in people.

Dr. J. T. Kent

GOOD PHYSICIAN

The physician's knowledge as to what he is doing, is his own, and the greatest comfort he can get out of it is his own. He need never expect that anyone will appreciate what he has done, or what he has avoided. The physician who desire praise and sympathy for what he has done, generally has no conscience. The noble, upright, truthful **physician works in the night;** he works in the dark; he works quietly; he is not seeking for praise.

Dr. J. T. Kent

HAY FEVER

Many a time have I seen hay fever **wiped out in one season** by a short-acting remedy, only to return the next season just the same, and perhaps another remedy will be required. As soon as the hay fever is stopped you must begin with **constitutional** treatment. There will be symptoms, if you know to hunt for them, that differ altogether from the acute attack.

Dr. J.T. Kent

HOMEOPATHY-NATURAL CARETAKER

The children that grow up under the care of the homeopathic physician will never have consumption, or

Bright's disease; they are all turned into order and they will die of old age, or be **worn out properly** by business cares; they **will not rust out.** It is the duty of the physician to watch the little ones. To save them from their inheritances and their downward tendencies is the greatest work of his life. That is worth living for. When we see these tendencies cropping out in the little ones, we should never intimate that they are due to the father or mother.

Dr. J. T. Kent

HUMAN MIND

We do not know half as much about the human mind as we think we do. We only know its manifestations. These little things belong to this **sphere of action of the medicine.** The one who knows the materia medica, applies it in its breadth and its length, and sees in it that which is similar.

Dr. J. T. Kent

IMPULSE TO SUICIDE

A *Natrum sulph.* patient will say, "Doctor, you do not know how I have to resist killing myself. An impulse to do it comes into my mind."

Dr. J. T. Kent

INJURY

Symphytum **follows** *Arnica* **well, if** pricking pain and soreness of periosteum remains after an injury.

Dr. H.C. Allen

KEYNOTES

If **keynotes** are taken as final and the **general** do not conform, then will come the failures.

Dr. M.L. Tyler

LACK OF REACTION

When not withstanding the **carefully chosen remedy** and the patient's faultless diet, the sick condition on the contrary, is not at all changed, the cause usually lies in want of **receptivity** which we must seek to remove either by repeated small doses or by medicines recommended for **deficient reaction.**

Dr. Boger

MODALITIES

The medicines that are similar in general have to be compared, as to **heat and cold.** In that way we get a list of those that are ameliorated by cold, and a list of those that are ameliorated by heat; and another non-descript list which are not ameliorated by either. That is the starting point, and we have to **divide and sub-divide** these, and so on.

Dr. J.T. Kent

When the symptoms seem to point out a particular remedy with which the **modalities however do not agree; it is only negatively indicated,** and the physician has the most urgent reasons to doubt its fitness; he should therefore seek for another, having the same symptoms.

Dr. Boger

NO SUBSTITUTE

No drug will do equally well for another curatively, while several may be more or less palliative, which is quite another matter.

Dr. M.L. Tyler

There must be no guess work in the study of provings. Every remedy must be used for its own symptoms, and for these, there is no substitute. If a remedy does not work, the homeopath can only examine the case a new and seek new symptoms and another remedy.

Dr. J.T. Kent

SMALL NUMBER OF HOMEOPATHIC PHYSICIANS

The capabilities of our materia medica are something wonderful, but they could be developed much more rapidly if a number of homeopathic physicians would make application of the materia medica with accuracy and intelligence, observing what they see and relating it literally.

At the present day, there is only a very small number of homeopathic physicians, that can come together in a body and say things that are worth listening to, a shamefully small number when we consider the length of time Hahnemann's books have been before the world.

Dr. J.T. Kent

POWER OF REMEDIES

Never think that homeopathy can cure everything; it cannot, but it can relieve even the incurable to such an extent that it is difficult to realize, at times its incurability.

Dr. M.L. Tyler

PREDISPOSITION TO DISEASES

Most of the substances that are used on the table as seasoning in foods will in the course of a generation or two be very useful medicines, because people poison themselves with these substances; tea, coffee, pepper; and these poisonous effects in the parents cause in the children a **predisposition** to disease, which is similar to the disease produced by these substances.

Dr. J. T. Kent

PRIMARY AND SECONDARY ACTION

In *Bryonia:* The urine is scanty and only exceptionally (or as I would express it **reactionally**) copious. We must remember that **every remedy has a dual action**. These two actions are termed **primary** and **secondary action**. I think that the so-called secondary action is only the reaction of the organism against the first or primary (so-called) action of the drug. For instance, the real action of *Opium* is to produce sleep or stupor, the reaction is wakefulness; of *Podophyllum*, *Aloes*, etc., the reaction constipation, and I think that the truly homeopathic curative must be in accord with the primary (so-called) effects of every drug in order to get the best and most radical cure, but if given for the secondary (so-called) symptoms, the primary ones having passed by, we should carefully inquire for all the symptoms which have preceded those symptoms which are present; and taking both past and present, let them all enter into the picture whose counterpart is to be found in the drug, which is to cure. Any other method is only palliative and not curative.

Dr. E. B. Nash

REAL CURE

While the patient himself with these deep psoric affections feels better, generally after the remedy, it will be months before his symptoms go away. He may say: "I feel better, but my symptoms all appear to be here. **I can eat better and sleep better." Then it would be unwise to change the remedy.**

Dr. J.T. Kent

REPETITION

It is a prime rule not to keep repeating your remedy when the **intervals** between aggravations of the disease are **lengthening.** This is an indication that the patient is improving.

Homeo. Recorder, Aug. 31

It has been frequently, the writers experience that, patients who are **slow to react** to remedies, have children with similar peculiarities and in such cases, **repeated doses are much likely to be needed.**

Dr. Hardy

High fever, great pain, great fear, strong fits of anger, or emotional excitement, shorten the **action of a remedy** and **indicate repetition.**

Dr. Pierre Schmidt

SINGLE SYMPTOM

No remedy should be given on one symptom. Study the remedy and disease thoroughly to ascertain if the two are similar to each other.

Dr. J.T. Kent

SMALL DOSE

If it be necessary in the case of a very sensitive patient, to employ the smallest possible dose and to bring about the most rapid result, one single olfaction merely, of **a single globule of the size of a mustard seed will suffice.**

Dr. Hahnemann

SPONGIA-VALVULAR DISEASES

I have never done better work with any other remedy in **valvular diseases of the heart than** *Spongia*.

Dr. E.B. Nash

SUFFOCATION-SLEEP OR WHEN AWAKE

When a patient goes to sleep, the cerebrum says to the cerebellum: "now you carry on this breathing a little while, I am getting tired." But the cerebellum is not equal to the occasion. It is congested, and just as soon as the cerebrum begins to rest the cerebellum goes to sleep, too, and lets the patient suffer; and in that way we get suffocation. The **cerebellum presides over respiration during sleep and the cerebrum presides over respiration when the patient is awake.** We might learn that from the proving of medicines if we never found it before.

Dr. J. T. Kent

SYCOSIS

Many of the ovarian or tubular symptoms that develop **during menses** are dependent on Sycosis.

Dr. H.A. Roberts

SYMPTOMS—TO BE STUDIED DEEPLY

All who do not perceive the difference between **symptoms predicated of the patient** and symptoms **predicated of the parts,** will see that, as only one symptom, with the rest of them. When he takes up a case and works it out in the repertory, he will use it as one symptom. Yet, that feature will sometimes rule out all the rest, because it is predicated of the patient and not predicated alone of his parts.

Dr. J.T. Kent

SYMPTOMS OF MIND

Hahnemann directs us to pay greatest attention to the symptoms of the mind, because the symptoms of the mind constitute the man himself. The highest and innermost symptoms are the most important, and these are the **mind symptoms.**

Dr. J.T. Kent

SYMPTOMS

When the symptoms have **been well gathered,** the case is as good as cured; it is easy then to find a remedy.

Dr. J.T. Kent

Basis of Great Achievements

One thing in homeopathy, taught in Hahnemann's organon is that, unless there are symptoms to **indicate the remedy, no great things should be expected from** the administration of the remedy.

Dr. J.T. Kent

I claim that he who prescribes, being guided by all the symptoms, will not and cannot fail, where a cure is at all possible. They are and must be our **infallible guides,** or Similia Similibus Curantur is not true.

Dr. E.B. Nash

A remedy fits a general condition when the symptoms of that general condition are found in the remedy. Remember that, it does so because all the symptoms agree.

Dr. J.T. Kent

The medicine that covers the symptoms is the one that will **change the economy** from an abnormal to a normal state, and digestion will become orderly, and we will have growth and prosperity in the economy.

Dr. J.T. Kent

THE SO-CALLED GERM DISEASES

They **cannot thrive in the blood or tissues, if the organism is not primarily sick** and affords a suitable soil for them. In health, immunity from germs is well known. When such an immunity is absent, health is likewise absent; under the circumstances, it becomes the duty of the true physician to **remove that susceptibility** of the organism to germs and other disease influences which constitutes the primary factor in **so-called zymotic diseases.**

Dr. Younan

TIME FOR A REMEDY

In acute troubles, if it is possible to wait the time through for the remedy, give it **very high at the close** of the attack, and you will be very likely to so **build up that constitution** so that the next attack will be much lighter.

Dr. J.T. Kent

TOTALITY OF SYMPTOMS

Any remedy, of course, which corresponds to the totality of the symptoms, is the remedy to administer.

Dr. J.T. Kent

VEGETABLE-MINERAL-REMEDIES

Unless the indications pointed strongly to one in preference to the other remedy, it might be well to try the **vegetable kingdom first.** The **minerals** are generally longer and deeper in their action, and would perhaps be **preferable in the more chronic the case.**

Dr. E.B. Nash

REMEDIES

ACONITUM NAP. (Routine habit): So called homeopaths have fallen into similar error, concluding that because *Aconite* did quickly cure in some cases having a high grade of fever, that therefore it was always the remedy with which to treat cases having high fever. **They even fell into the routine habit** of prescribing this remedy **for the first stage of all** inflammatory affections, and follow it with other remedies more appropriate to the whole case further on.

Dr. E.B. Nash

ACONITUM NAP.: From fright, vertigo comes on, or fainting; trembling; threatened abortion, or suppressed menstruation. **Jaundice may be induced by it,** and become chronic. There are other remedies for fright, prominent among which are *Opium, Ignatia, Veratrum album*, etc. Now, in regard to the dry, cold air, no remedy has more prominently acute inflammations arising from dry, cold air. **Nineteen out of twenty cases of croup arising from exposure to dry, cold air will be cured by** *Aconite*.

Dr. E.B. Nash

ARSENICUM ALB.: It makes little difference what the disease, if this **persistent restlessness** and especially if great **weakness is also present,** don't forget *Arsenic*.

Dr. E.B. Nash

AURUM MET. (Emotions and intelligence): We shall see that the **affections are interior,** they are covered with a cloak, they are his innermost and are hidden from inspection; but the **understanding is the outermost garment,** it surrounds and hides his affections, just as does the garment he wears over the body hide the body. The affections that *Aurum* resembles are those like, into the very **innermost nature** of man.

Dr. J.T. Kent

AURUM MET. (Gloom and despair): The Aurum patient is plunged into the deepest gloom and despair. Life is a burden, he desires death. Suicide dwells constantly in his mind. **In men,** I have observed it oftenest in connection **with liver troubles. In women, with womb troubles,** especially when enlarged, indurated or prolapsed. In both these cases, the result, so far as local conditions are concerned, seems to be from repeated attacks of **congestion to the parts, which ends in hypertrophy.**

Dr. E.B. Nash

AVENA SAT. (Tonic): It is prescribed in 10 to 20 drop doses of the tincture in a little water for its alleged tonic effect; numbness of the limbs, as if paralysed, is said to be symptom. It does seem to quiet the nervous system and bring about sleep; it like-wise relieves nervous headaches and fatigue most assuredly; it is to be preferred to the powerful coaltar drugs so constantly abused.

Dr. R.F. Rabe

BELLIS PER.: In old workmen, laborers, and the over **worked and flagged,** *Bellis perennis* is a princely remedy.

Dr. Burnett

CALCAREA CARB. (Sad girl): It is a strange thing to see a bright little girl of 8 or 9 years old taking on sadness, melancholy, and commencing to talk about the future world, and the angels, and that she **wants to die and go there,** and she is sad, and wants to read the bible all day. That is a strange thing; and yet *Calcarea* has cured that.

Dr. J. T. Kent

CALCAREA CARB. (Sphere): It has no such tearing down nature in it. It does not establish inflammation around foreign bodies and tends to support them out, but causes a **fibrous deposit around bullets** and other foreign substances in the flesh. It causes tubercular **deposits to harden** and contract and become encysted.

Dr. J. T. Kent

CALCAREA CARB. (Modality): Suppose the patient always avoided warm things and much clothing, and wanted the cold open air, and still had a dozen key-notes, you would find every time that **Calcarea would fail.**

Dr. J. T. Kent

CALCAREA SULPH: Most inveterate catarrh of the nose has been cured by this remedy.

Dr. J. T. Kent

CALCAREA SULPH. (Kidney): This is a valuable remedy for catarrh of bladder, with copious yellow pus. It has cured chronic inflammation of the kidney.

Dr. J. T. Kent

CAUSTICUM (Throat): Dryness of the mouth and throat; rawness of the throat, must swallow constantly on account of a sensation of fullness in the throat, a nervous feeling in the throat. This is often a **fore-runner of paralysis.**

Dr. J. T. Kent

CIMICIFUGA RACE. (Change of symptoms): A woman will come to you with **one group of symptoms** today and may come back to you with an entirely different **group in a couple of weeks.**

Dr. J.T. Kent

CINA: When there is a **papillae** on the tip of the tongue, the child has worms, *Cina* is the remedy.

Dr. Edwards

COCCULUS IND. (Paralytic stiffness): It is entirely **without inflammation.** It is a sort of a paralytic stiffness, a paralysis of the tired body and mind. In *Cocculus*, headaches and backaches, pains and distress are present. A man will stretch out his leg on a chair and **he cannot flex it until he reaches down with his hands to assist.**

Dr. J. T. Kent

COLOCYNTHIS (Sphere): You will **seldom find this** medicine indicated in strong, vigorous, healthy people who have suddenly become sick.

Dr. J. T. Kent

CUPRUM MET. (Convulsions): During the progress of the labour, the **patient suddenly becomes blind.** All light seems to her to disappear from the room, the labor pains cease, and convulsions come on, commencing in the fingers and toes. When you meet these cases, do not forget *Cuprum.*

Dr. J. T. Kent

CUPRUM MET. (Discharges): The individual has become debilitated and worn out with excitement, but this discharge barely kept him alive. He has gradually grown weaker, but he has kept about because he had a **discharge.** It has furnished him a **safety valve. If stopped suddenly, convulsions will come on.**

Dr. J. T. Kent

CUPRUM MET.: A drink of **water seems to flow through the bowel with a gurgle.**

Dr. J. T. Kent

DULCAMARA (Habitual cold taking): Every experienced physician must have met with many cases where, for a time he felt unable to cope with the case because of his inability to reach the constitutional state that underlies this **continual tendency of taking cold.** So, he puzzles, for a long time, and prescribes on the immediate attack and palliates it.

Dr. J. T. Kent

FERRUM MET. (Haemorrhage): Woman suffers much from haemorrhage from the uterus, especially **during and after the climacteric period.**

Dr. J. T. Kent

FERRUM MET. (Feeble constitution): She is **feeble,** she suffers from palpitation and dyspnoea, she has great weakness with inability to do anything like, work, she feels that she must lie down, yet the face is **flushed.** This is called a pseudo-plethora.

Dr. J. T. Kent

FERRUM MET.: (Green sickness): "Ferrum will be found of great value when the symptoms agree-in that wonderful anaemic state called, "green sickness," that comes on in girls **at the time of puberty** and in the years that follow it. There will be almost **no menstrual flow, but a cough will develop,** with great pallor. So common is this sickness among girls that all mothers are acquainted with and dread it.

Dr. J. T. Kent

GELSEMIUM SEMP. (Erysipelas): May not have produced erysipelas, it will stop the progress of the disease in a few hours, and the patient will go to a quick recovery. If we master thoroughly the Materia Medica, **we do not stop to see, if a remedy produces certain kinds of inflammation, etc., but we consider the state of the patient.**

Dr. J. T. Kent

HEPAR SULPH. (Leucorrhoea): The **leucorrhoea** is so copious that she is compelled to wear a napkin, and the napkin, I have been told by women who have been cured by

Hepar, are so **offensive** that they must be taken away and washed at once because the odour permeates the room.

Dr. J. T. Kent

HYOSCYAMUS NIG. (Sensitive to pain): When the patient is ill natured, unreasonable and complains beyond all reason, **in rheumatism,** or any other disease, a few doses of *Hyoscyamus* 3x will surprise you very pleasantly.

Dr. Cuthburt

IGNATIA (Deranged mind): A sensitive girl, though she would not let anyone, but her mother knows of it, falls in love with a married man. She lies awake in nights, sobs. She says, "Mother, why do I cannot keep that man out of my mind."

Dr. J. T. Kent

IGNATIA (thirst of special nature): Thirst, when you would not expect it. Thirst during chill, but none during the fever, if she has a feverish state.

Dr. J. T. Kent

MEDORHINUM: The husband's histories give the cause, and this remedy will cure.

Dr. J. T. Kent

17. SYMPTOMS AND HOMEOPATHY

Dr. E.B. Nash was the **first** physician to lay **sole** emphasis on symptoms in selection of remedies. He believed in administering **single** dose of a **single** remedy. He was even **against** alternating two medicines. He mentioned about **one alternation** (Rhus tox. and Hyoscyamus) in his life for which he felt **guilty**. He also claimed of achieving wonders with a single dose in **chronic** and difficult cases.

But in general practice, dependence on **symptoms only** does not lead us to such success. Then, what was the **secret** which he **could** not or **did** not reveal!

The fact is that in practice he **established** coincidence between the **sphere and the symptoms of** the remedies and the diseases.

Regarding Sepia, it is told that it works on a particular **tooth**. Then it is seen that **Phosphorus** cures the toothache of **washerwomen**. These are indicators of the relations between sphere and remedies.

We can see the method of **Nash's** working in the **arrangement** of remedies in his 'Leaders' on the **basis** of spheres. His 'Trios' also indicate sphere and category e.g. Digestion, Flatulence, Heart, Liver, Delirium, Convulsion and Women remedies.

Dr. Kent has also emphasized the role of sphere. He finds that **every remedy has a sphere** of its own.

Dr. **Hahnemann** could cure 183 cases of Typhus without a single failure **purely on this basis.** Almost **each** of his patients was having some **difference in symptoms.**

Dr. **Farrington** observed that **Rhus tox.** cures **Lumbago irrespective** of its general symptoms.

Actually, our failures or hit and miss phenomenon in Homeopathy is due to our wrong approach to the system.

We have been told at several occasions about the **nature** of medicines and the diseases; and also **advised** to consider the **stage** of the medicine and disease to get favourable results.

Dr. **Nash or Dr. Kent must be having** complete picture of drug **personalities** whereby they could match them with the patients by their **appearance.** Dr. Nash speaks of **"Tell Tale Face"** in this context only.

The fact is that we are always inclined to follow some easy method - even when it is wrong or incomplete. This leads us to disappointments.

We find today that some people are getting used to depend on **Repertories.** This is a **mechanical** process and Homeopathic prescribing **needs** deep study, intelligence and wider understanding. Repertories **can not** prepare us to present a picture of personalities in medicine and acquaint us with various other **aspects** like potencies, danger points, acute or chronic stages, fast and slow medicines, patch up remedies, etc.

Then sometimes **modalities** also mislead us. **Phosphorus** may be thirstless, **Psorinum** may be hot, also **Silicea** may be hot sometimes.

All round vigilance is the keynote for good results in Homeopathy.

Lastly, we all know that much still remains to be explored when Homeopathy can become a mathematical science in certainty.

∎

18. THE NATURE OF A DISEASE AND HOMEOPATHY

It is told in the name of **Dr. Hahnemann** that a homeopath has nothing to do with the **name** of a disease and a patient has nothing to do with the **name** of a medicine!

It is merely an exhibition of ignorance.

The name of a disease simply **comprises** of some symptoms grouped together. It enables us to **comprehend the picture of sickness** in a moment. If such way is **defined** by the profession, it means that the ulterior motive is not fair and honest and may aim at keeping the patient in dark and confusion **in the name of symptoms.**

Similarly, the name of the remedy **should be** made known to the patient. It should not at least denied in the case of persons who are educated or have some interest in the system or one to know the name for any other reason.

In the present state of affairs that homeopathy is practically practiced on **individual** basis and no **norm** has been established. It is all the more necessary that the name of remedy is not **concealed**.

Some of our pioneers may have followed the practice of not telling the name of medicines at some time in their life and it might have **valid** reasons for their doing so.

Firstly, it may be that the Homeopathic remedies were not so freely available as we get today. **Dr. Nash** used to make many potencies on his own **potentizer.**

Secondly, they followed the system of a **single dose of a single remedy** and wanted to wait and watch the results. In such situation, if the patient has free access to the medicine, he has the chance to repeat the doses even if **unwanted.**

Dr. Kent has indicated about such situations. But the conditions today have changed. We do not always meet such **conscientious** physicians and the **people** on the other hand are being used to bulk consumption of remedies. We find people **asking** for one month's remedy or two month remedies and such occasions are seen **increasing.**

Any way, we should not be touchy in telling the name of the remedy if the patient is so interested.   ■

19. "NEAR SPECIFICS" IN HOMEOPATHY

The concept of near specifics was first given by **Dr. Hahnemann.** It means that the nature, sphere, stage and symptoms of a remedy **coincide** with these aspects of the disease.

Actually we try to establish this **match** in each case to the maximum extent possible, if favourable results are desired. This is actually done in **individual** cases.

But there are certain conditions which are **generally** found in the **'world of sickness'** and there are certain conditions which **commonly** cover such situations. **It is here** that we get the benefit of the near **specifics** that stand the clinical testimony in majority of cases.

Such efforts in this direction were meant to simplify our way to medication.

The method was devised to save us from confusions and complications on the one hand and maintain our scientific process on the other.

But people of profession deviated from this path and started **mixing** many remedies working on a **particular** sphere and declaring them as **"approved specialities"**. This was the result of a **commercial attitude** which **threw**

homeopathy away from the principles on which it was established.

This is a cheap way of reaching a common man directly by manufacturing agents. They have won the physicians' confidence on the basis of financial allurements.

Thus, a huge gap takes place between those who really practice scientific homeopathy and those who join hands with people who deviate.

As far as common mass is concerned, it is not enlightened. People look at homeopathy as a mere system which 'LABELS' it bottles with name 'Homeopathic Remedies.' Quality of medicines and scientific selection or prescriptions has no meaning for them. If they get relief they think they are cured! If there is no relief they think that the system has failed to cure them!

If homeopathy has to progress and prevail, people have to be enlightened and educated, and the physicians have to be conscious, honest and deep in studies, and also not narrow in their approach.

At the moment, the system is in bad shape. It has derailed from its scientific way and aims, as are religious, political parties and other organizations in search of easy gains.

Let us hope for real specifics to revive and survive.

■

20. PROVINGS AND CLINICAL TESTIMONY IN HOMEOPATHY

The concept of homeopathy is based on its **'proving'** on healthy, conscious, educated and enlightened individuals who can feel and express the **language of body** when it reacts to the drugs in potency on body, mind and emotions.

This started with scientific **explorations** and the aim was to make it a **mathematical science in certainty** where only one straight line could be drawn between two given points.

But practical difficulties and **limitations** were seen in this process. **Firstly,** every individual differs from the other in one way or the other on physical, mental or emotional level and it is natural that the 'provings' made on one will **differ** sometimes **greatly** and at another time totally with the other.

We also find some 'drugs' to **react** generally in a more or less **similar** manner and in this **group**, we find the so called **'near specifics'** which we establish after **'Clinical Testimonies.'**

Then, over long years of experiences, and conscious observations, we gathered some **features** that are equally important to affect a good cure. **Under this topic** we find our **relationship** of remedies, complementaries, inimicals, antidotes or dangerous remedies and then particular times when some remedies **act better.** Repetition of remedies in **certain potencies** in different cases, acute or chronic remedies are **also** important for studies and consideration.

There are also situations when provings **cannot form** the basis. **Sickness** of pregnant ladies, very old men, infants and children and many other phases of life have to be dealt on the basis of our best assessment and judgement from different **angles** where experiences, foresight and clinical testimonies guide us in selection of remedies.

But if we consider all the aspects in view, in the context of drug effects in general, homeopathy may be considered as **near to safe** as compared with **Allopathy where** potency does not minimize the crude effects and little more quantity can make the case suffer.

The need of the hour is to standardize the quality of manufacturing and lay stress on judicious and careful selection of remedies with certain 'norms' that may be established.

■

21. WHETHER

- Homeopathy cures permanently.
- Homeopathy is safe without any precondition.

It is claimed that cures through homeopathy are **permanent**. It may be said as **ridiculous**. Any sickness or disease occurs **due to** some reason or deficiency. **If** a man is cured by **certain** remedy, the same circumstances or conditions can again **cause** the sickness. There is nothing in the world which can work as a **"safety valve."**

Homeopathy — if used rightly or judiciously can affect a **natural** cure. It means that it can **regulate** the system wherever faulty.

If used wrongly or incorrectly, it may **mask** or camouflage the original symptoms. Actually, symptoms are the **language** of the body meant to express the place and type of **irregularity** or deformation occurring at any time. We have to understand and recognize it **before** this process damages the body.

Homeopathy helps us to locate and find the sickness in the **primary** stage, through the symptoms in the **body and mind.** It is special boon of this 'pathy' for the mankind. If the medication is not 'correct' the voice of the system is likely to be **masked** and the process of damage may continue without any **'signal'** to us.

This is the way, Homeopathy harms us and such situations, as **Dr. Kent** points out, are likely to be **most dangerous on earth.**

If a pain originates from heart, and a process of damage is taking place there and a patient is given simple **painkiller,** then it may be that the pain subsides and the patient **sleeps forever.**

It is true with any or every 'pathy'— when it is **incapable** of finding the cause and sphere of the ailments as also the stage of the disease and prescriber **wrongly**—the results are likely to be damaging and dangerous.

So, we cannot **claim** Homeopathy to be sage in all conditions and all the time—we use it, **unless** used properly with all cautions required by the system. **Dr. Kent** has given many wise suggestions and directions in this regard. **He has mentioned** that **Ferrum met.** can be dangerous in certain stages, **Kali carb.** also needs to be careful in particular stage, and then **Pulsatilla** prepares the ground for **Silicea** is to work nicely. We also need to know about **'Patch up'** remedies in certain stages.

In nutshell, caution or vigilance is the keynote to save the patient from danger and render him a natural cure.

22. COMPARATIVE MERITS OF HOMEOPATHIC SYSTEM OVER OTHERS

- **A single** dose in potency can work wonders.

- **It does not** require its doses to be necessarily continued for long to complete certain course with regard to quantity or time.

- **It works** too fast, rather instantly if correctly prescribed and the quality of medicine is of standard.

- **The discontinuation** of medicine at any stage or missing any dose does not have any harmful effect **as in case** of antibiotics in Allopathy.

- The medicines are easy to store and they are not subject to **expiry** of time like medicines in other systems.

- **The medicines** are **easy to use** and not aversive for the patient of any age or condition.

- **A drop** of medicine can be put on the tongue even in case of a patient in serious condition **when swallowing** anything is not possible.

- **A household kit** can be maintained by conscious and educated people who can use the medicines **at odd hours** and difficult situations under direction of their family physician.

- **It does not** require the cumbersome process of costly and inconvenient **tests and examinations** every now and then.

- **At the present** there are more than one hundred **'near specifics'** where we are saved from confusion and get almost sure results.

- **Many of the emergencies** and acute painful stages can be met with the system **at little cost** and very quickly, eg. toothache, earache, colic, gastritis, dysentery, diarrhea, cystitis, whitlow, sciatica, excessive uterine bleeding, painful menses, painful or bleeding piles, arthritic attacks, epileptic fits, cramps and convulsions etc.

- Ailments of infants, children, old men, and pregnant women are special fields of the system.

- **Difficult and chronic cases** like aphthae, migraine, fistula, high blood pressure, diabetes, kidney stones, gallstones, dyspepsia, gout, tonsillitis, sinusitis, marasmus, psoriasis and other skin diseases, various types of allergies are **better manageable** under homeopathy than with other systems.

- **It is true** that a disease like tuberculosis has not been conquered by the system but it helps in the primary stages and sometimes checks the progress of the disease and **cures it in the initial stage.**

- **In general day-to-day problems** like acute allergies, headache, sleeplessness, bodyaches and joint pains, where patient feels obliged by taking painkillers or sleeping pills or antiallergic drugs, **the system** can enable the people to seek the cause and remove the factors responsible for **frequent attacks** by increasing resistance and **regulating the system.**

A **homeopath** has to accept that certain **emergencies** which require **immediate surgery** or sedatives are **out of** **the scope** of his system. But he has to know his own **exclusive sphere** fairly and deeply whereby he can help majority of cases of various types **to save** high expenses, going through difficult processes and **facing** complications and confusions.

We should all know that no system is perfect but if we can understand the comparative advantages or merits and demerits of each we get a better choice of our advantage.